NEAL'S YARD REMEDIES

Homoeopathy

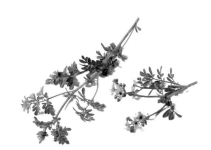

NEAL'S YARD REMEDIES

Homoeopathy

Principles • Sources of remedies • Modalities

Mental symptoms • Emotional symptoms

Physical symptoms • Raw materials • Dosages

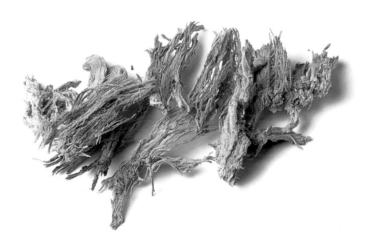

Rebecca Wells

AURUM

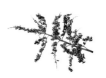

Author's Acknowledgements

I would like to thank Alison Wells and Gideon Berman for all their wonderful support and advice, Romy Fraser for giving me the opportunity to write the book, and Tom Mettyear for his initial introduction to the joys of homoeopathy and his continued enthusiasm that has touched my life enormously. *RW*

First published in the UK in 2000 by
Aurum Press Ltd
25 Bedford Avenue
London WC1B 3AT

Text copyright © Neal's Yard Remedies, 2000
Artwork copyright © Haldane Mason, 2000
Copyright © Haldane Mason, 2000

ISBN: 1-85410-709-7

A HALDANE MASON BOOK

Conceived, designed and produced by Haldane Mason, London

Editorial Director: Sydney Francis

Managing Editor: Beck Ward

Editor: Ben Keith

Art Director: Ron Samuel

Designer: Zoë Mellors

Picture Research: Ben Keith

Colour reproduction by Emirates, Dubai

Printed in Hong Kong

Picture Acknowledgements

Cover photograph by Amanda Heywood. All photographs by Joff Lee, with the exception of the following: **A–Z Botanical Collection:** /Anthony Sweeting 21, /Oleg Kosterin 49, /Adrian Thomas 51, /Bob Gibbons 57, /Dan Sams 64, /Malkolm Warrington 69; **Mark Warren:** 14, 17; **Mary Evans Picture Library:** 9; **Natural History Museum:** 27, 63, 78; **NHPA:** /Robert Erwin 8 & 90, /Stephen Dalton 25, /Daniel Heuclin 42, /Bill Wood 96; **OSF:** /Michael P. Gadomski 53; **Rowan McOnegal:** 28, 29, 35, 36, 37, 52, 54, 61, 82, 87, 89, 101, 102; **Science Photo Library:** /Hattie Young 13, /Carl Schmidt-Luchs 50, /Dr Morley Read 68, /Eye of Science 71, /Seth Joel 73, /Charles D. Winters 85.

Contents

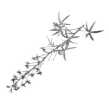

Foreword

Homoeopathy was the principal motivation behind the setting up of Neal's Yard Remedies in 1991, which is why it is particularly exciting to be introducing this book – the third in the series. Knowing that Becky was a popular practitioner as well as the manager of our busy shop in Elgin Crescent, we asked her to try writing the monographs for the natural medicine course. The result was excellent. In fact, it was so good that we realized that the material could be used to form the basis of the long-awaited homoeopathy book.

In the early 1970s I studied homoeopathy, and for three main reasons: first, I wanted to be able to look after myself and my new baby; second, I was intrigued by the notion that something could be more powerful the more subtle it becomes – 'less equals more' defies our modern materialistic understanding of the world; and third, I loved the remedies themselves, with their strange sounding names and even more extraordinary descriptions of the indications.

Homoeopathic medicines took priority at the first shop in Neal's Yard in Covent Garden, and although herbs and essential oils quickly found their places on the shelves, the homoeopathic principles have remained a fundamental part of the company. It is a system of healing that can only become more popular in a society that is becoming increasingly aware of its environment. More importantly, because the remedies are made from the substance that can cause the disease, homoeopathy can provide solutions to many new health problems, as well as being uniquely adaptable to social, climatic and environmental changes or disasters. In addition, enormous quantities of remedies are made from very small amounts of their raw materials. When you consider the number of lavender plants needed to produce a small bottle of the essential oil, it is worth appreciating that from the sting of a single bee it would be possible to treat each and every person in the whole world with the remedy Apis (page 24). It is a highly practical system for the future, and this makes it accessible to everyone, wherever they live.

At a time when public health services are coming under increasing pressure and their quality of service is being more closely scrutinized, learning how to look after ourselves can give us a great sense of empowerment. We increasingly want to know what is going on with our own bodies and we want to be able to be more in control of our health. Indeed, as our environment changes – from the food we eat to the clothes we wear – the one thing we can and should be most aware of is our health. This is, of course, what we try to encourage people to do at Neal's Yard Remedies.

I established the business in 1981 so that people could purchase natural remedies. I also provided expert assistance to help people choose the remedy to match their type. From studying homoeopathy I learned about people and how they function and gained an understanding of patterns in illness, in individual symptoms and in behaviour. One becomes an expert at observing people. When one starts to place oneself in the context of society one can spot trends and can start to appreciate the laws of cause and effect. This might seem irrelevant, but in a situation where there is a shop full of people, each wanting to choose the right remedy, it is vital to know not only which remedies treat which illnesses but also to have an understanding of which remedies suit which personalities. This will become clearer the more you delve into the descriptions of the remedies in the Materia Medica section of this book.

Becky has been working behind the counter at our shop in Elgin Crescent for several years, and with calm confidence she has assisted many customers to recognize the remedy most suited to their needs. This has contributed to the excellent reputation and success enjoyed by the West London shop. She is now a full-time practitioner but for me it is her experience in answering customers' queries which makes this such an invaluable book as she is so familiar with what people want to know.

There are currently so many books available on natural medicine that it is impossible not to wonder if there is room for another. I believe that there is. This book not only contributes an excellent series of remedy pictures to enjoy for their own sake but it also provides a background for simple and effective prescription. This book will help you to understand homoeopathy, how it works and how to pick your own remedy. It is a book we are proud to add to our collection, and I know it will be invaluable to our customers and staff, as well as to homoeopathic practitioners who like to recommend to their patients an informed and intelligent guide to treatment.

Romy Fraser
Neal's Yard Remedies, London
January 2000

Introduction to Homoeopathy

There are many different kinds of alternative and complementary health practices available today. This abundance of choice can leave us feeling overwhelmed and confused. Informed choices are vital, however, as part of the responsibility that we now have – and need – to understand our own health and the health of our families.

Homoeopathy is a holistic health practice, treating the person as a whole when diagnosing the problem, rather than taking the illness out of its personal context and treating it in isolation. This book aims to give a better understanding of homoeopathy and its philosophy through the detailed yet straightforward accounts of some of the more commonly used homoeopathic remedies. The accounts, described in the Materia Medica section, illustrate the peculiarities of each remedy to make it easier to administer in accordance with the peculiarities of the patient.

Homoeopathy is a complex subject and can be confusing when applied for the first time. An understanding of the homoeopathic process and philosophy behind it is vital for effective prescription, making any introduction to homoeopathy an important part of the whole.

The remedies mainly come from natural sources. Poison ivy, for example, is used when making Rhus tox.

The best introduction to homoeopathy is to see a professional homoeopath, who is trained to provide constitutional treatment (this will be discussed later). These visits will help the new patient to learn about homoeopathy, and they will also help strengthen the immune system and increase vitality. The patient will then be able to apply the remedies at home when needed.

Self-knowledge is an important and exciting thing, but respect for different healing methods and how these are used is important in the safety and understanding of our health and general well-being.

WHAT IS HOMOEOPATHY?

Homoeopathy comes from the Greek word *omeos*, meaning 'similar', and *pathos*, meaning 'suffering'. This literal translation indicates one of the fundamental aspects of homoeopathy: the principle of 'like cures like' – something causing imbalance in the body being used to restore balance. This was first introduced by the ancient philosopher Hippocrates, but brought to life and developed by a

German doctor, Samuel Hahnemann, in the late eighteenth century.

Hahnemann was a highly respected physician who became disillusioned by the medical practices of the time. He was dismayed by the lack of curative response to the methods that were used and the inadequate philosophy of these practices.

THE LAW OF SIMILARS

Hahnemann's first observation of 'like cures like' came as a result of reading an article on the uses of Peruvian bark (the source of the homoeopathic remedy known as China – page 48) for the treatment of malaria. Hahnemann felt that the author's explanation of why the bark was such an effective remedy was unsatisfactory, so he decided to take small quantities of the Peruvian bark himself to discover, by first-hand observation, if it had any effect on a healthy person.

Hahnemann made a note of all the symptoms that he felt after taking the bark, and experienced what we know today to be the symptom picture of China, namely: numbness of his extremities, intermittent fever, a hard, small pulse, anxiety and mental stupor. He found that the symptoms would disappear after a few hours only to reappear if he repeated the dose. What he was experiencing were all the symptoms that are associated with malaria. Hahnemann was, in fact, producing the very symptoms that Peruvian bark was prescribed to cure!

Samuel Hahnemann (1755–1843), an eminent German physician, was the founder of homoeopathy.

PROVING

As a result of these extraordinary observations, Hahnemann realized that if he could discover the effects that other substances had on a healthy individual, then he could also discover what these substances would help to cure. He began to experiment on himself, using an array of substances and studying existing accounts of accidental poisonings, thereby broadening his range of remedies. He called this method of establishing the effects the substances had on healthy people 'provings'.

Hahnemann's work led to a comprehensive, detailed understanding of the homoeopathic remedies. This needed to be matched by a detailed understanding of the patient; the individual and unique symptoms of each patient became of vital importance in diagnosing the illness.

Occurring naturally in our bodies, Calc fluor is used to treat chilblains and toothache.

Due to the subtle nature of homoeopathic medicine, tablets should be stored away from direct sunlight and strong-smelling substances.

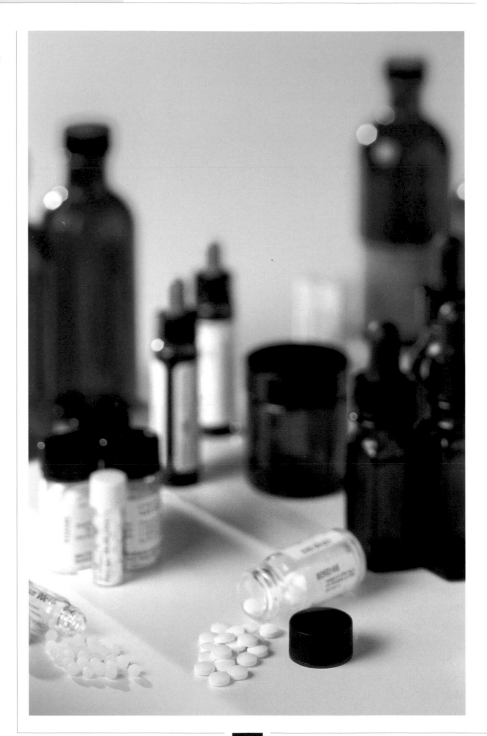

POTENTIZATION

The remedies were, however, still capable of producing side-effects. Hahnemann found that by diluting the substances further, these side-effects disappeared. He also established that if the remedies were shaken vigorously during the dilution – a practice known as succussion – this released the previously dormant energy of the substance, making the remedies more potent. Each remedy was diluted to such an extent that in some cases there were barely any actual material substances left. Hahnemann believed that what existed after this dilution and succussion was the transference of the energy belonging to the original material into the new, neutral material.

THE VITAL FORCE

The concept of energy, or vitality, is an important one in homoeopathy. Just as it is necessary to understand the vitality of the remedy, so it is to understand the vitality of the patient.

We all have a life-force or energy running through us, which, quite literally, keeps us alive. This force maintains balance, enabling our bodies to adjust to the constant change required in our lives. In homoeopathy this is known as the 'vital force' and is a similar concept to the 'chi' and 'prana' of Eastern medicine.

Just as nature has its own regulating mechanism so to do individual people. We are unable to understand the exact meaning of this, or to locate it

scientifically, but we are aware of the flux that we experience in our own energy state. The homoeopathic concept is that when our vital force is out of balance, then our bodies and minds produce symptoms such as colds, rashes and depression as an expression of this disharmony. The energy held within the remedies helps to stimulate the energy of the vital force, thereby rebalancing at this fundamental level.

SUSCEPTIBILITY

The issue of how vulnerable different people are to disease and ill health is an important one. Some people have amazingly robust constitutions, rarely succumbing to illness, regardless of their lifestyle. Others are susceptible to every illness imaginable, even if they exercise daily and eat a balanced diet.

Many factors determine the strength of your constitution. Genetic inheritance is an important one. Illnesses and weaknesses that run through families are often passed down through generations, and many people find that they have similar health patterns to other family members, such as a tendency to asthma or eczema. Others may find that there is one area that is always affected when experiencing disharmony in their life, such as headaches or a skin irritation.

Rue, from the Greek reuo, means 'to set free'. It is used in the remedy Ruta for the treatment of sprains.

We all respond in different ways according to our own constitution. Homoeopathic remedies can help strengthen and change these patterns, thus altering the patterns of our susceptibility. By doing this, homoeopathy can prove vital in the prevention of disease as well as being curative in specific cases of illness.

Repeated stresses in our environment that put pressure on both our physical and emotional selves can also weaken our constitutions. The concept of a maintaining cause – a continuous stress that creates no room for change – can damage our ability to rebalance. It is important that we address these issues as part of our increasing commitment to health.

The common red onion is the source of Allium cepa, a highly versatile remedy.

ACUTE AND CHRONIC DISEASE

It is important to define an illness as either acute or chronic as this helps patient and practitioner alike to recognize the level on which it should be treated.

Acute illnesses are self-limiting; that is, they have a defined duration, which usually includes an incubation period, a showing of the illness and then a time in which to convalesce. Death can also be the final stage of an acute illness, however, so it is always important to consider professional advice when treating an acute condition.

A chronic illness occurs over a longer period of time, with a gradual increase of debility, often displaying many different symptoms as the illness develops. The length of a chronic illness is largely unknown, and 'guesstimates' will vary depending on the nature of the disease and the constitutional strength of the patient.

The question of suppression – alleviating a presenting symptom without looking at the underlying cause – is an important one here. The body shows physical and emotional symptoms as a sign of disharmony. If acute illnesses constantly arise and are continuously suppressed by medicines without looking at the causation, then the underlying imbalance may ultimately produce a more chronic condition. This is not to say that self-help treatment is inadvisable, but the process of homoeopathy can be particularly effective, supportive and empowering in the treatment of acute illnesses that are understood. The remedies do not act in a suppressive way, but instead allow the body to heal and rebalance itself as a whole.

THE REMEDIES AND HOW THEY ARE MADE

The selection and description of remedies that are available in homoeopathy are collectively known as the 'Materia Medica'. There are many Materia Medica books available to the homoeopath, listing all the findings from

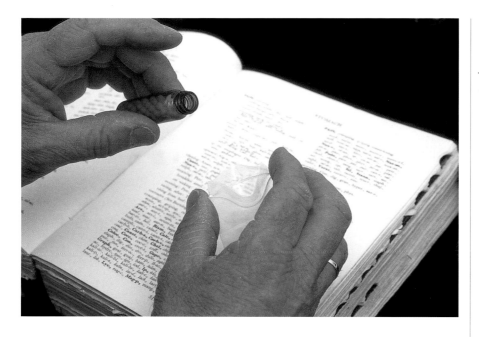

Remedies are dispensed in tablet form after the patient's symptoms have been carefully observed.

the original provings. The number of remedies is vast and is increasing all the time as different substances become available and new provings are carried out. There are 62 remedies included in this book. There is also a table of External Materia Medica on page 14.

Intricate knowledge of the remedies is increasing due to recorded clinical use, not to mention improved communication in the homoeopathic world.

The remedies are mainly sourced from nature – plants, animals and minerals – although some synthetic substances are also used. It is important to note that there is no cruelty to animals in the making of homoeopathic remedies.

When buying homoeopathic medicines, remedies of different potencies are available. Potency refers to the amount

of times that the remedy has been diluted and shaken, and therefore what strength or amount of energy is contained within it. The more a remedy has been shaken and diluted, the stronger it is.

There are two main scales used in the making of remedies and these are represented at the end of the remedy name, e.g. Pulsatilla 6x or Pulsatilla 6c. The '6' represents the number of times that the remedy has been diluted and shaken; the 'x' or 'c' represent the proportions in which the substance has been diluted.

The source of the remedy is first steeped in alcohol for a period of time. This is known as the 'mother tincture'. The 'x' is a representation of the decimal scale of dilution. This means that one-tenth of the mother tincture

EXTERNAL MATERIA MEDICA

External Materia Medica are plant extracts. They have not been 'proved' so are not proper homoeopathic remedies, but they can be very effective when applied directly to the affected area. They come in two main forms: oil-based creams and tinctures. Tinctures are made by steeping the relevant plant in alcohol for a long period of time to extract its healing properties, then diluted with water before application.

Arnica A cream or a tincture that is applied to reduce swelling and bruising after an injury. It is important that the cream is not applied to an area where the skin is open from a cut or wound.

Calendula In its cream form it is particularly soothing for skin irritations, such as eczema, burns and nappy rash. As a tincture it can be applied in a diluted form as an antiseptic lotion for routine cuts and grazes.

Comfrey It is used as a cream to promote the healing of stubborn cuts and sores; it also helps scar tissue to form correctly. However, because of its speed in healing wounds care must be taken to ensure all wounds are cleaned thoroughly to eliminate any infection. Comfrey's affinity with broken bones means that the cream is also effective in reducing swelling and promoting the healing of fractures.

Euphrasia The tincture is diluted and used to bathe sore and irritated eyes. Use two drops diluted in half a cup of boiled, cooled water and apply. Be careful never to put the undiluted tincture directly in the eye.

Hypericum and Calendula This combination has powerful antiseptic properties as either a cream or a tincture, helping to promote rapid healing in cuts and wounds. It is also used to reduce profuse haemorrhaging from open wounds and is excellent for injuries to parts rich in nerves.

Hypericum and Urtica These two plants combine to form a cream that soothes the pain and irritation of minor burns.

Rhus Tox and Ruta This cream relieves injuries to the ligaments and muscles.

Stellaria Made from the herb chickweed, it is a cream used to relieve itchy irritations, such as chicken pox and eczema.

Thuja A tincture that is usually applied undiluted to treat warts and verrucae. It should be used three times a day for at least one month and is best used in conjunction with internal homoeopathic remedies.

is taken and diluted into a further nine-tenths of alcohol and then shaken. This is called the '1x' potency. One-tenth of this dilution is then taken and diluted into a further nine-tenths of alcohol and then shaken. This becomes the '2x' potency, and so on. The 'c' is a representation of the centesimal scale of dilution. This means that the mother tincture is diluted by taking a one-hundredth of it and diluting it into ninety-nine parts of alcohol and shaking it, creating the '1c' potency. One-hundredth of this solution is again diluted into a further ninety-nine parts of alcohol and shaken, creating the '2c' potency, and so on. The more the source is diluted, the greater the strength of the remedy, therefore 6c is stronger than 6x and 200c is stronger than 6c. Remedies that do not naturally dissolve in water are ground for many hours so that they become water-soluble.

HOW TO TAKE A REMEDY

When the required potency has been achieved, the remedy is administered via a carrier; this is usually in the form of tablets or granules made from lactose or sucrose. For first-aid prescriptions, it is better to use lower potencies, although the remedy potencies can go very high, and many homoeopaths use remedies that have been diluted thousands of times. The remedy should be placed under the tongue and left to dissolve. It is important that the remedy is taken in a clean mouth, so no eating or drinking for about twenty minutes before or after taking the remedy is advised. Due to the subtle nature of homoeopathic remedies, they can be antidoted by very strong smells and substances such as eucalyptus, camphor or peppermint products—alternative toothpaste can be obtained from most health food shops.

Only one remedy should be taken at any one time, and the appropriate remedy can be selected only after close observation of the patient's symptoms. One tablet or a few granules is equal to one dose. After taking the initial dose it is important to observe any changes of symptoms as the remedy starts to work. Always stop if there are signs of improvement and start again if the symptoms return, or change the choice of remedy if the symptoms change.

Side effects are rare when using the remedies, but if any one remedy is taken too often, symptoms of it may sometimes start displaying or 'proving'. Moreover, it is not necessary to take the remedies over a long period of time as they act as stimulants to the body's own healing mechanism.

THE HOMOEOPATH

Unprejudiced observation is crucial when taking a case as assumptions can lead to false information that may

Experiments with Peruvian bark led Hahnemann to investigate the uses of homoeopathic medicine.

mask any important features. The emotional state of a patient is of great significance: if you have a friendship or a relationship with your patient, then it is often very difficult to look at their condition from an objective viewpoint, especially if the psychological aspect of their condition is important. This makes it difficult to prescribe for close friends, and is a good reason to consult a homoeopath on a professional basis.

Homoeopaths will tend to ask detailed questions, including those that may often seem irrelevant, such as what type of weather or food the patient prefers, as well as specific responses to the patient's condition. The medical history of the family is also important. This depth and detail of questioning is vital in the holistic aspect of finding the right remedy for the whole person.

The art of finding the right remedy can be a difficult one. The remedies can often reveal old imbalances that have been masked by conventional medicine or an unknown suppression of symptoms. The period of treatment usually corresponds to the period of illness. Monthly visits to a homoeopath are generally advised as a starting point.

During the early stages of treatment from a homoeopath, remedies will often be administered in a higher potency.

Carbo veg – a remedy taken from charcoal may seem an unlikely medicine but it is excellent for asthma and indigestion.

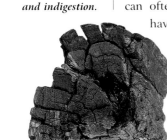

It is common for the patient to receive just two or three tablets to help stimulate the body's natural healing mechanism, aiding rebalance and healing over several months. This is a dramatic move away from any conventional medicinal practices, which tend to use repeated and multiple doses of medicine over long periods of time.

After taking a constitutional

Phosphate of potassium – one of the body's tissue salts that is used to make the remedy Kali phos.

remedy from your homoeopath, the symptoms can sometimes get worse briefly – known as a 'healing crisis'. This reaction is often perceived as a good sign because it shows that the body is starting to speed up its natural healing processes. Other symptoms that occur may include colds, diarrhoea, feelings of tearfulness or even a return of old symptoms. These will not last long, however, and are all signs that the body is starting to cleanse itself.

THE MATERIA MEDICA

The way in which the remedies are discussed and explained may seem quite peculiar on first sight. The accounts of the remedies are known as 'remedy pictures'. These pictures usually cover all aspects of the human condition, from mental and emotional

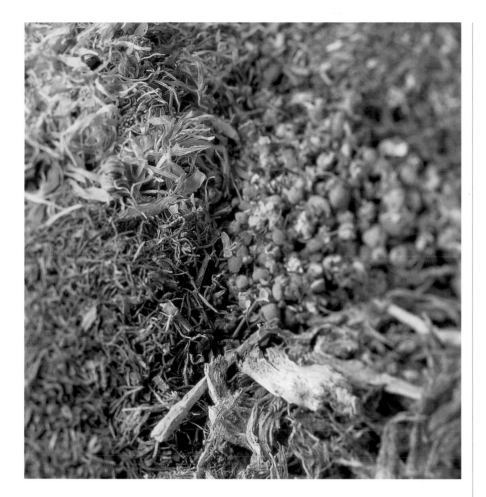

Homoeopathic remedies are prepared from plants, minerals and animals.

states to the physical one. The remedies have their own characters or 'essences', and the person who needs a particular remedy may be described as a remedy 'type': we may talk about a 'Nux vomica type' or a 'Calc carb character'. The symptoms of the remedy can also be characterized, such as a 'Belladonna headache' or an 'Ant tart' cough. The more information received about a remedy, the easier it is to understand its picture.

AILMENTS & REMEDIES

This final section contains descriptions of each ailment, with the symptoms appropriate to the relevant remedies to help you choose the right one.

Homoeopathy is a subtle and effective form of treatment when used in the right way. This book aims to provide a greater understanding of how it works and to encourage confidence in the remedies and the benefits that this amazing system of medicine brings.

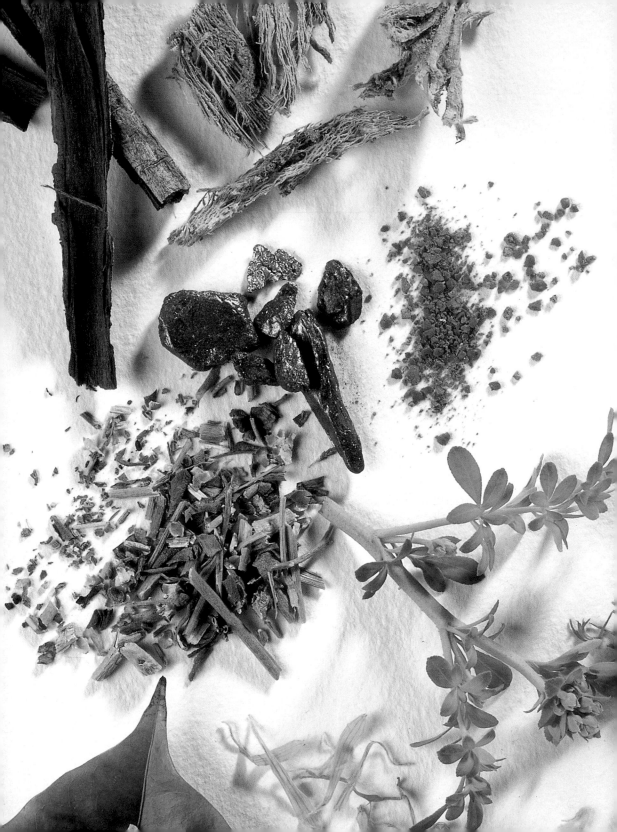

The Materia Medica

This section forms the heart of the book, containing portraits of 62 commonly used homoeopathic remedies. Each remedy portrait has been divided into three parts: a description of the material or plant from which the remedy is made, a mental and emotional symptom profile, and, finally, a description of the physical complaints associated with that remedy. Each remedy has a unique symptom picture, so it is important to look at all the aspects of each remedy for a greater understanding of how it can be used effectively. Many of the remedies have a variety of uses, the most common of which are listed alongside their descriptions.

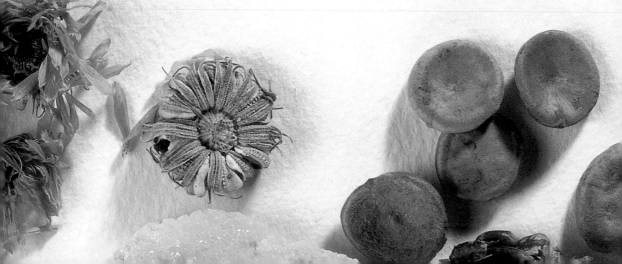

Aconite

FULL NAME
Aconitum napellus
(Plant family:
Ranunculaceae)

COMMON NAMES
• Monk's hood
• Wolf's bane
• Helmet flower
• Friar's cap

The tall upright plant of Aconite is a member of the buttercup family and is often found on mountain slopes in shady areas. It reaches about 4–5 feet (1.2–1.5 m) in height and is topped with an asymmetrical array of vibrant blue flowers. They are shaped like a hood or cap, hence one of Aconite's most common names: Monk's hood.

Below the ground, the root is similar to a horseradish root in size and colour. This has led to the root being eaten by mistake, as a result of which many of the poisonous indications of the plant have been discovered. Aconite is known to be an extremely deadly substance, and accounts of its powerful action have been documented. It is said that hunters living in the Alps would dip their arrows into the fresh juice of Aconite as a deadly weapon against wolves, giving it its other name of Wolf's bane. Historical accounts of the Burmese war also talk of Aconite being used with devastating results.

From the tragedy of the accidental poisonings, Aconite has become one of the most effective homoeopathic first-aid remedies in the Materia Medica, giving joy, however, rather than grief.

MAIN INDICATIONS

MENTAL AND EMOTIONAL

Throughout the Aconite picture we find that the human organism is affected very rapidly – this is particularly evident in Aconite's use as a poison, when death can occur within two or three hours of consumption. The sudden onset of symptoms, therefore, is very distinctive of this remedy's homoeopathic picture. Even the most robust people are affected quickly. It is this suddenness that causes one of the main emotional pictures of Aconite – that of fear! This fear is an intangible one: the patient will fear darkness, bed-time, ghosts and some will even predict the exact time that they will die. There is rarely calmness with this remedy; restlessness prevails, escalating to panic and terror. In fact, Aconite has been used very successfully in labour when the mother becomes scared and panicked, convinced that there is no way that she will survive the birthing process. The Aconite emotional state may reflect a terrifying experience that happened previously – for example, the suddenness of a heart attack, a car crash or the experience of labour may leave the patient feeling uneasy and emotionally traumatized long after the actual event.

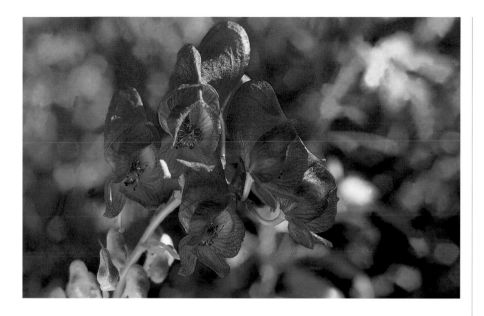

PHYSICAL

On this level, the reaction of Aconite is also sudden, acute and often violent. One of the most common uses of this remedy is at the beginning of a cold after exposure to dry, cold winds. The body will go into a violent, inflammatory state after the initial chill or shock. The respiratory centre will be affected by a short, dry, croupy cough that causes wakefulness during the night, inducing the patient to sit bolt upright. The face often becomes hot and flushed, with a look of anxiety, or you will find that one cheek is pale and the other red. The heart can be pounding, especially during a fever, and there is often a sensation of tingling, prickling and warmth, usually in the hands and feet. The throat often feels inflamed, raw and sore. Restlessness and a burning thirst, particularly with a high fever, accompany all this. Most of the symptoms of Aconite are worse at night, especially around midnight. If there is haemorrhaging, the blood is bright red and the pains will be extremely intense and unbearable.

The Aconite patient will usually be quite a strong, robust person, which makes the sudden onset of illness more of a shock to the system.

The Aconite picture will go almost as quickly as it appeared, so it is therefore important to catch it in the initial stages before another remedy picture comes in sight. To reiterate, the sudden onset is all-important.

Common Uses

- Colds • Sore throats • Sudden shock
- Panic attack • Fright • Bronchitis
- Croup • Earache • Fever

MODALITIES

Worse: *sudden emotions such as fright and shock; being chilled by dry, cold winds; cold sweats; noise; light; teething; night-time; sitting up in bed*

Better: *open air; resting; warm perspiration*

Allium cepa

FULL NAME
Allium cepa
(Plant family:
Liliaceae)

COMMON NAME
• Red onion

Everyone is familiar with the way in which our bodies react when we are chopping onions: eyes stream, noses run profusely and we want to rub at our eyes to relieve the stinging. If this picture is kept in mind, it becomes easier to understand the main uses for this homoeopathic remedy.

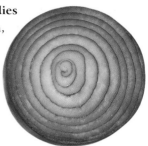

MAIN INDICATIONS

MENTAL AND EMOTIONAL

Allium cepa patients feel dull in the head and may fear that they will never recover from their illness.

PHYSICAL

All mucus discharges are greatly increased in this remedy picture. The nose feels as if it is burning and the left nostril is usually affected first, before the right one. The burning, acrid discharges from the nose make the upper lip red, raw and incredibly sore. The eyes feel tender and burning and water profusely, but the tears are bland and do not affect the face, unlike the nasal discharge. The opposite occurs with the remedy Euphrasia (page 54), where the nasal discharge is bland but the tears will burn.

Allium cepa is an excellent remedy for colds and hay fever, especially when the colds usually start as a result of cold, wet weather and the hay fever is worse in August. Profuse sneezing is usually the first tell-tale sign, triggered by the smell of flowers or peaches, and possibly worsening when the patient enters a warm room. The nose begins to feel raw and sore, then the eyes start to water. The cold may move down to the larynx, where the patient feels a splitting, tearing sensation, which often makes them hold their throat to relieve the pain. Walking into cold air can trigger a tickle in the throat that sets off coughing. There is a tendency to feel much worse at night and in the evening because the body is too warm. The head may feel congested and throb and the eyes are often sensitive to light. Allium cepa is a good remedy for colic in children when they have to double up to try to relieve cutting, tearing pains.

Patients are also averse to cucumbers, but, unsurprisingly, they crave onions.

MODALITIES

Worse: *warm rooms; smell of flowers and peaches; eating cucumbers; cold, wet, windy weather; autumn; spring*

Better: *fresh air; moving around*

Common Uses
• Hay fever • Colds • Tickly coughs
• Headaches

Ant tart

Antimony is another of the poisons used in homoeopathy. It is odourless and comes in the form of white powder or clear crystals. This made it a fine tool for murderous acts in the same way as Arsenic (page 30). Medicinally, it was used in small quantities as an emetic to encourage vomiting, although obviously this could be a very dangerous, even deadly practice. The dangerous effects of Antimony are harnessed in this remedy to establish a positive homoeopathic use.

FULL NAME
Antimonium tartaricum

SOURCE
• Antimony – potassium tartrate

COMMON NAME
• Tartar emetic

MAIN INDICATIONS

MENTAL AND EMOTIONAL

The patient feels exhausted: there is great lethargy, drowsiness and pitiful moaning, especially from children. Patients will also suffer extreme irritation, particularly when they think that they are being watched or are about to be touched. Frightened by the symptoms, however, some children want to be held, usually in an upright position, and may cling tightly to their parents, while others try to find solitude, just wanting to be left alone.

PHYSICAL

The Ant tart patient produces a great deal of white, watery, slimy mucus, especially from the lungs. Any rattling and bubbling from the chest when the respiratory system is suffering can be extremely noisy. The patient's weakness and lethargy make it difficult to cough up much of this mucus, which then builds up rapidly, restricting breathing and making it uncomfortable to lie down. The entire body becomes extremely pale and sickly, with sunken eyes and a bluish pallor to the face. Cold, clammy sweating is typical; hands and feet feel like ice, but warmth makes the symptoms feel worse, so patients prefer having the windows open and the bed covers off. They should also avoid drinking fluids as this may cause vomiting.

Ant tart is a useful remedy when the patient has continuous attacks of bronchitis and repeated colds, or a cough that has been present since their time of vaccination. It can also be effective against chicken pox when the rash appears slowly and the cough is as described above.

Ant tart should be used when any exhaustion suffered is particularly acute.

Common Uses
• Bronchitis • Colds • Cough
• Chicken pox

MODALITIES

Worse: *heat; anger; eating; drinking; touch; being looked at; lying down; autumn; spring; very early hours*

Better: *coughing up mucus; sitting up; cold*

FULL NAME
Apis melifica

SOURCE
• Honey bee

Apis

This remedy captures the essence of the honey bee. It is usual for the whole body of this extraordinary insect to be used in the making of the remedy, not just the contents of the venomous sac.

Bees are sensitive and restless creatures, which toil unrelentingly in an almost predetermined way for the good of the hive and their queen – hence the expression 'busy as a bee'.

MAIN INDICATIONS

MENTAL AND EMOTIONAL

The mental and emotional picture of Apis is somewhat predictable if one thinks about bees themselves. Apis types are fidgety, restless and even slightly nervous. They can show feelings of hypersensitivity and are occasionally aggressive – think of the bee that is interrupted in its work! Their hard work is often fruitless and unproductive, characterized by clumsiness and a certain number of silly mistakes. Socially, Apis patients may act in an ungainly and awkward manner, perhaps laughing inappropriately at other people's misfortunes, for example, only to find that no one else is amused.

Apis types hate to be alone and demand attention. However, when that attention is offered, perhaps in the form of affection, they reject it. There is also a concept among Apis patients that empty spaces must be filled, whether it is a gap in conversation or the physical void left by the death of a loved one. They are given to flirting a great deal, and sex can play an important part in their methods of communication. They enjoy movement and dancing, and often dream of flying or travelling.

PHYSICAL

As with Aconite (page 20), the onset of illness in an Apis patient is often quite violent, becoming rapidly worse. The pain with Apis is fiery, stinging and burning, and the affected area will look and feel very hot and red. Sometimes the pain may feel as if a red-hot needle, very similar to the sensation of a bee sting, has pierced the affected area. In fact, not surprisingly, Apis is one of the primary first-aid remedies for bee and wasps stings.

Inflammation and oedematous swellings often occur as the fluid rushes to the affected part. Many symptoms of Apis are due to fluid 'filling the spaces' – i.e., fluid in the testes, ovaries and pleural cavities.

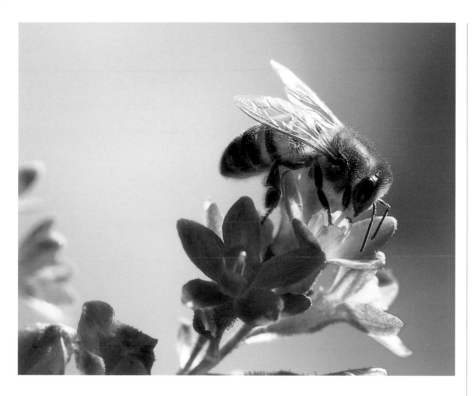

(Incidentally, under a microscope oedematous tissue looks very similar to the intricate cavities of a beehive.)

Any swelling may have a shiny appearance or a pale, waxy look, and there is often a stiffness and tension in the affected part, although movement isn't aggravating in the same way as Bryonia (page 37), as the fluid becomes redistributed. A finger may leave an indentation when it has prodded a puffy area.

Apis is a useful remedy for cystitis when the last few drops of urine sting and smart and the patient must strain to pass water. There is a definite lack of thirst with this remedy, especially when hot, although there may be a craving for milk, taken in small sips. The patient feels incredibly hot-blooded and cannot tolerate heat in any form.

Many complaints will start on the left-hand side and spread to the right; the pain can move around the body.

Symptoms are much worse between three and five o'clock in the afternoon, and anything cool will give enormous relief. Touch of any sort is rarely tolerated; even touching the hair can feel painful.

Common Uses

• Insect bites • Abscesses • Allergies
• Cystitis • Mumps • Styes

MODALITIES

Worse: *heat; touch; after sleeping; mid to late afternoon; pressure; lying down*

Better: *being cold; moving about and changing position; sitting upright*

FULL NAME
Argentum nitricum

SOURCE
• Silver nitrate

Arg nit

Alchemists knew silver nitrate as *lunar caustic* in medieval times. It was used then as it is now: for the treatment of epilepsy and cauterizing wounds. Silver nitrate comes in the pure form of colourless, odourless crystals, which are acutely light sensitive, turning grey or black upon exposure and turning the skin black on contact. It is an extremely effective disinfectant but it is highly poisonous if consumed, causing inflammation, especially of the mucous membranes, violent cramping, convulsions and eventual paralysis.

MAIN INDICATIONS

MENTAL AND EMOTIONAL

The Arg nit person is nervous, hurried and impulsive. There is a huge lack of coordination on both the emotional and physical levels. Weakness prevails in the mental process, and a loss of mental ability occurs as the emotional state takes over. Patients feel overwhelmed, excitable and apprehensive. Anticipatory anxiety predominates: if there is a project to be completed or a public performance or examination looming, patients will feel extremely nervous and anxious about failing. They know that their brainpower is diminishing and their memory loss is becoming increasingly acute.

Rationality can also fade as the Arg nit patient starts to react too quickly, rather than stop and think – so all reasoning goes out of the window. Worse still, this irrational behaviour may lead to impulsive ideas, such as jumping in front of a train or off a bridge. The underlying irrationale of Arg nit is 'but what if . . . ? What if I did jump – what would happen then?' These patients can envisage entire crazy scenarios that lead on from one 'what if' to another, then another, until they are actually reacting to something that isn't happening at all.

Arg nit patients suffer from a great many fears, which are often expressed physically by an upset stomach or diarrhoea. They are terrified in crowds or situations where they feel trapped and claustrophobic. Heights present a particular problem, and their legs may give way. Alternatively, they may fear that tall buildings will fall down on top of them. Even bridges and spiral staircases are frightening, as are any viewpoints from which it is possible to look down, below or through. This is a great remedy for fear of flying, which combines all the usual fears of the Arg nit patient in one.

Arg nit types need lots of company and get very nervous being in the house, or even leaving the house, on their own. Nervous break-downs are common within this remedy; nothing seems easy and even the most simple, everyday tasks become an enormous ordeal – patients simply cannot cope with the day ahead of them. A strange symptom that Arg nit patients have, which in many ways expresses their internal situation, is the delusion of being a soda bottle. It represents the feeling that some part of them is about to explode because the stress is just too great.

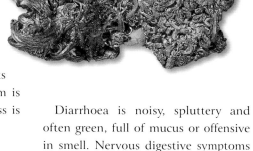

PHYSICAL

As with Pulsatilla (page 88), Arg nit patients need a great deal of fresh air, and they like to sleep with the windows open or walk outside. Cold food and drink can also help, although their craving for sweet foods can aggravate the digestion, especially if they eat too much. A nursing child can even be affected if the mother eats a lot of sweet things and then breast-feeds.

Extreme anxiety accounts for much of the general digestive disorder. Abdominal pain is rife, together with very unpleasant gaseous and bloated feelings. Patients may experience a great deal of flatulence and belching, which are very loud yet don't seem to relieve any discomfort.

Diarrhoea is noisy, spluttery and often green, full of mucus or offensive in smell. Nervous digestive symptoms are much worse after eating.

Anxiety also manifests itself in heart palpitations, together with vertigo and fainting, although, strangely, the palpitations are felt mainly on the right side of the body, away from the heart. The legs tremble from weakness.

Many of the symptoms are accompanied by vomiting, sometimes whole mouthfuls, quite suddenly. Headaches feel congested and full, and normally start during any mental effort; they are relieved by tight bandaging or pressure to the head.

Common Uses

- Anxiety • Diarrhoea • Flatulence
- Belching • Fainting • Headaches

MODALITIES

Worse: *emotion; anxiety; warm rooms; sugary foods; hot food or drink; confined spaces*

Better: *fresh air; hard pressure; cold food or drink*

FULL NAME
Arnica montana
(Plant family:
Compositae)

COMMON NAMES
• Leopard's bane
• Mountain tobacco

Arnica

Arnica can be found growing just below the snow line at high altitudes and is most common in Switzerland, northern Germany and the Andes in South America. It is related to the daisy and grows to about 6 inches (15 cm) in height. The flowers are bright yellow – like the daisy's – and have a slightly dishevelled appearance, as if they have been bashed around by driving winds. The root is woody and has a peculiar smell of apples. Arnica prefers to grow in soft, rich, moist soils made from decaying matter – ground that would cushion a fall. It has traditionally been used in the Andes as an infusion for those who have been badly injured after a mountain accident.

MAIN INDICATIONS

MENTAL AND EMOTIONAL

Arnica is one of the best known and most effective first-aid remedies available to us. There are very few accidents, bumps, scrapes and shocks that do not initially benefit from a dose of Arnica.

To understand the emotional picture of Arnica you just need to think of someone in a state of shock. There is a huge reaction of withdrawal, as if they have been knocked out of their physical body and a wall has been built around them. Arnica patients usually dismiss any suggestion that they are unwell or hurt, they are averse to being touched, because of the pain, and they will be irritable, sending away anyone who tries to help. They have a feeling of detachment from themselves and others.

Numbness can be present and a feeling of contrariness – these patients don't know what they want or who they are. Arnica is a great remedy for jet lag when these feelings can be strong and any sense of time is lost. Apathy and weakness are often apparent.

There is a darkness to this remedy, often showing itself through dreams of dark forms and hallucinations of mutilated bodies. Arnica patients may have a strong fear of death, but not as strong as in the picture of Aconite (page 20).

28

PHYSICAL

Arnica is the remedy for injuries, accidents, traumas and shock. It is particularly relevant where there is bruising or any tearing or breaking down of blood vessels. With haemorrhages it is invaluable when trying to arrest bleeding anywhere in the body. This remedy really is a master healer at any time of crisis, aiding the body to recover at a faster rate.

There are numerous ways in which Arnica can be used, and it is often beneficial to administer it in those situations where a trauma can be anticipated. For example, taking a dose of Arnica before a visit to the dentist can reduce the amount of swelling or bruising that may occur. Taken during and after childbirth, Arnica is a fantastic healer, especially if there is a large amount of haemorrhaging. In cases of concussion, whether there is a fracture or not, Arnica will help to reduce swelling after any injury.

There is often increased sensitivity. The body feels sore, bruised all over, and the muscles really ache. The bed can feel too hard, causing restlessness and making sleep impossible, and any jarring of the bed will be unbearable.

Many of the discharges experienced can be offensive, with sweat, stools and breath smelling of rotten eggs. A strange symptom of Arnica is that eruptions appear symmetrically on the body, such as a boil on each cheek or thigh or acne equally on either side of the face. Many of these eruptions may appear after a trauma.

The head can feel extremely hot in contrast to the body, which is cold. This can cause many differing types of headache. For example, the head can feel as if a nail has been driven into it, or as if the brain as been shattered into a thousand pieces. Despite all this, any blow to the head should initially be treated by the remedy Arnica, whatever type of pain it is the patient is suffering from.

Arnica is an exciting remedy to discover and may be used at home safely and effectively as an excellent first aid treatment for everyday mishaps.

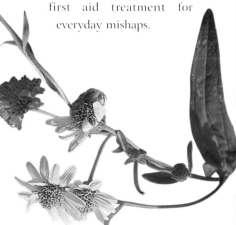

Common Uses

- Shock • Injury • Accidents • Trauma
- Haemorrhage • Bruising

MODALITIES

Worse: *motion; rest; lying on the affected part; damp; cold*

Better: *lying down; open air; cold; washing; uncovering; changing position; sitting upright*

FULL NAME
Arsenicum album

SOURCE
• Arsenic trioxide
• Sulphide of arsenic

Arsenicum

There are many poisons in the homoeopathic Materia Medica, but none is as famous as arsenic. If one were to consider murder then the administration of arsenic would be high on the list for undetected efficiency. From the Borgias in the fifteenth and sixteenth centuries to the present day, there have been innumerable deaths from this seemingly harmless, odourless, colourless substance.

Arsenic was so widely used in the reign of Louis XIV that the whole era was known as 'The Age of Arsenic'. Death is not a certainty, however, as there are many different levels of tolerance. Indeed, it is a known practice for people living at high altitudes to use arsenic to aid breathing. Toxicity is dependent on the size of dose, the form of administration, where it enters the body and the susceptibility of the subject. In the horse-racing industry small doses of arsenic are administered to give the horses sleek, shiny coats and to keep them on their toes for races. It is also given to turkeys to increase levels of breeding and to prevent disease, although it can prove fatal if a treated turkey is consumed at a later date.

From the results of arsenic poisonings, we can develop a homoeopathic picture of one of the most widely used remedies in the Materia Medica.

MAIN INDICATIONS

MENTAL AND EMOTIONAL

There is great anxiety and restlessness present in this remedy. Even when ill, and despite extreme weakness and exhaustion, an unexpected restlessness is present. Anxiety about health is especially evident.

Arsenicum characters are the ones who corner you at a party to tell you about their latest affliction. The prospect of cancer is particularly in their thoughts, and they have a constant worry that their body will let them down. The combination of anxiety and restlessness creates a great deal of vulnerability, but this is counter-balanced by a sense of extreme order in their lives. Things need to be neat and tidy, socks need to match and pictures need to be straight, otherwise they will feel nervous.

People also play a big part in the lives of Arsenicum types. They need a great deal of support and are always better in company, especially when ill. They will create a strong network of friends and acquaintances to give themselves security. They can be great leaders, enjoying the fact that people need them for decision-making and group efficiency.

Their dependency on others can make them seem like human leeches. They can be helpful and kind, but usually for their own gain and security. They tend to know what they want and make sure they can get it, manipulating people where necessary.

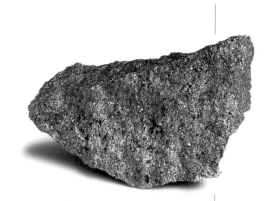

PHYSICAL

Arsenicum patients feel extremely chilly, but the chill is external – inside the pains are burning and fiery. All their symptoms are much better for hot things and they will desire warm drinks, lots of warm bedding and hot applications. During a headache the head will feel very cold but the body will be warm.

Restlessness is conspicuous, with extreme prostration and exhaustion that is completely out of proportion to the patient's complaint. Every reaction is expressed in an extreme way.

There are a lot of complaints associated with the digestive tract, and Arsenicum is one of the main remedies for food poisoning and gastroenteritis. The diarrhoea is frequent but comes in small amounts, with burning pains in the stomach and when passing stools. Anything that is eaten will be vomited immediately, although there is a thirst for small sips of water.

Arsenicum is a great remedy for asthma, especially if an attack has been triggered from emotional stress. The onset is usually very sudden, with extreme weakness and restlessness. Patients are very fearful and cannot lie down, but have to prop up their heads with pillows. The attacks will usually happen after midnight, when patients will suddenly sit bolt upright with a suffocating cough that produces an expectoration like whipped egg. In addition, burning pains will be felt in the lungs. Warm, sweet milk may ease the attack.

Any colds experienced produce fluid in the form of corrosive discharges that stream from the nose, making it sore and ulcerated. Sneezing is profuse.

The skin can be dry, scaly and unhealthy looking. There may be a desire to scratch until it bleeds. Ulceration occurs here as well, both on the skin and in the stomach. Malignancy may be present in later stages.

Common Uses
- Diarrhoea • Gastroenteritis
- Food poisoning • Asthma • Anxiety

MODALITIES

Worse: *cold drinks; food; after midnight; lying down*

Better: *company; being warm; moving around; raising the head; cold air – especially for headaches*

FULL NAME
Aurum metallicum

SOURCE
• Gold

Aurum

Gold has great meaning in human society: it is the symbol of wealth and success. Athletes run for it, wars have been fought for it and, in many ways, the beauty of this substance has led to much destructive behaviour, which reflects nothing of its original qualities. Nevertheless, gold still holds world-wide fascination. It is a shiny, bright and enticing metal, and, symbolically, it can be used as a remedy when the light and beauty represented by gold has disappeared from a person's life, only to be replaced by the more empty values that we have given to it in our society.

MAIN INDICATIONS

MENTAL AND EMOTIONAL

There is a dark, bleak feeling with this remedy, where the love for life seems to have been lost. Aurum patients feel weary and depressed and lack confidence in their abilities, perhaps with a desire to die. They can become so desperate that suicide is a real possibility for them. They feel no enjoyment of anything or anyone. Work, family and things that used to bring joy and happiness to them no longer do so. They are pessimistic, gloomy and full of self-condemnation and guilt. Despite hard work and the ambitious goals they set themselves, the burden of feelings such as a deep sense of failure and a neglect of responsibilities will prevail. These failures, whether real or imagined, are hard to cope with.

Initially, Aurum types find it difficult to connect with the world on any deep, emotional level; in fact, they can feel quite separate from their surroundings and find it painful to form close friendships, often throwing themselves into their work instead – hence their enormous sense of ambition. This means that they have very little outlet for expressing their true feelings. They often show great generosity and kindness that does not actually involve any emotional commitment on their part. The lack of reward for this attempt to connect with people can lead to feelings of resentment that they try to bury. They can have an immense sense of logic that tends to overrule negative thoughts. It is this suppression that can push them towards deep depression.

The Aurum character can feel better as the sun goes down, but sleep is often disturbed and patients may moan and call out in their sleep as vivid nightmares take over. Night-time is also when many of their physical pains intensify, leading them to feelings of despair. Any attempt to overcome their feelings of gloom can lead them to express themselves through anger and irritability. This can seem hurtful and irrational to others but their intention is not to be cruel – it is their only outlet.

The people who figure in the lives of Aurum characters will often be shocked when they observe any state of collapse. As a result, patients are determined to try particularly hard not to let anyone see their true feelings until the last possible moment.

PHYSICAL

Aurum has an affinity with the heart – one of the emotional centres of the body. There is a weight on the chest as if the heart has stopped, and this sensation is as if the heart is thumping too violently. Palpitations and breathlessness may be experienced when moving around, alongside watery swellings of the lower limbs and ankles. High blood pressure is also common. Aurum patients can get waves of flushing heat throughout the body, as if the blood is about to burst out of their veins, with rushes of blood to the head.

They can suffer with aching, boring bone pains, which travel down the longer bones, especially in the legs. The pain can be so severe that it feels as if the legs are broken. The joints are also affected: the cartilage around the joints can swell and become extremely painful, especially at night, preventing sleep or waking the person up. This pain will either create depression or make any mild depression more severe.

The destruction and breakdown described on the emotional level are evident on the physical level too. Ulceration is common in many areas of the body. The nose can be painfully ulcerated, with the ulcer producing a foul-smelling discharge and causing an

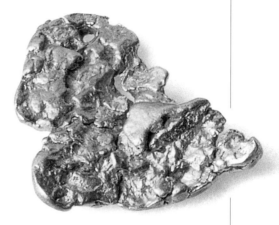

obstruction that makes breathing difficult. There is ulceration of the gums and they may start to look red and swollen, with the breath smelling putrid as a result.

Headaches are violent, with tearing pains in the bones as if the skull is bruised or fractured. The eyes can be incredibly sensitive to light, with soreness and pressure of the eyes and eyeballs that disturb vision. The bones around the eyes are also painful.

Common Uses

• Depression   • Heart palpitations
• Headaches

MODALITIES

Worse: *night-time; cold air; mental exertion; guilt; resting; winter*
Better: *warmth; movement; walking; summer*

Belladonna

FULL NAME
Atropa belladonna
(Plant family:
Solanaceae)

COMMON NAME
• Deadly nightshade

Belladonna is found throughout Europe, where it flourishes in chalky, shaded areas. It grows at an incredibly rapid rate, almost to the height of an average human being in just one season. The stem is tall and hairy, with a reddish-purple tinge, and the leaves are dark green. The flowers hang like large bells and are a pinky-purple colour. It is the berries that are most appealing: succulent and shiny, they look like small cherries that are sweet to taste; children adore them at their peril. As with Aconite (page 20), Belladonna is another viciously acting poison, which has been repeatedly used for the disposal of unwanted persons. It was especially favoured by the Lithuanians in the seventeenth century: if debts failed to be delivered, Belladonna was promptly administered to the debtor's drink!

The name Belladonna means 'beautiful woman' and comes from this remedy's use – primarily in Italy – as eye drops because it helped pupils dilate, supposedly making women more alluring.

MAIN INDICATIONS

MENTAL AND EMOTIONAL

With Belladonna we find an acuteness of all the senses. There is great excitement, movement and an intensity of reaction. Many of the symptoms are sudden and violent, which can often lead to a hallucinogenic state with delirium and an intense fever. Belladonna patients may have terrible nightmares, which cause them to kick, strike, bite and pull people's hair. The phrase 'an angel when well, a devil when sick' is particularly appropriate for Belladonna types. These patients often react to the slightest thing: noises, jarring of the bed or light, and, therefore, they feel better for rest, silence and darkness.

Fear is pronounced, and Belladonna patients will imagine that they see strange things – especially black dogs and gallows – even though their eyes are closed. They may also have a fear of water. All these symptoms can appear and disappear very quickly.

PHYSICAL

In an acute situation, Belladonna can be indicated very early on. Patients will have hot, red skin, and the pupils will be dilated and glassy, like 'beautiful women', as mentioned above. The face will be flushed and the pulse will be throbbing, making the patient agitated and very restless. The mouth and throat are usually dry, and the patient

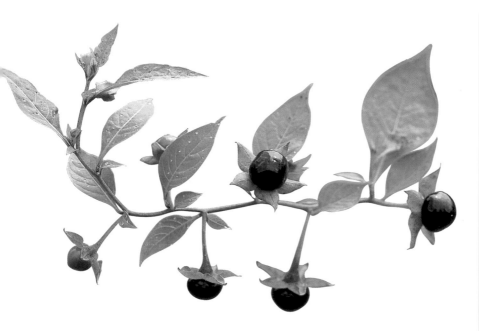

Worse: *sunshine; getting too hot; 3 p.m.; draughts around the head; cold wind; a hair cut; not being able to sweat; light; noise; jarring touch; movement letting parts of the body hang down (e.g., a hand); company; lying on painful side; bright, shiny objects; after midnight; bending the head forwards*

Better: *resting in bed; light bed covers; bending the head backwards; warm, dark rooms; standing or sitting upright*

has a craving for lemons or lemonade, although there will be a strong aversion to water. Heat, redness and dryness are all usually present. Local areas around the body can be greatly inflamed, as well as burning-hot and tender when touched.

Belladonna types are much worse if exposed to cold air, which may even provoke a sudden, violent reaction. Any headaches are pounding and throbbing, and there is a sensation of turmoil in the brain; even washing or cutting hair can bring on these symptoms. Clutching the head during a headache or bending the head backwards are common tactics with these patients to try to relieve the pain. Silence and darkness will help.

Belladonna is a particularly useful remedy for sunstroke headaches when

the sufferer has become far too hot. In tonsillitis, when the throat is dry, red, burning and inflamed, Belladonna is again an invaluable remedy. The patient wants to swallow but liquids do not go down well. The tongue may look red and textured like the skin of a strawberry.

A Belladonna picture can appear anywhere in the body, bearing in mind that it is at its most acute at 3 o'clock in the afternoon. The most important symptoms to look out for are dry heat, redness and pain.

Common Uses

- Abscesses • Boils • Bronchitis
- Chicken pox • Earache • Fever
- Headaches • Mastitis • Mumps
- Sore throat • Sun burn

COMMON NAME
- Daisy
- Bruisewort

Bellis perennis

The common daisy is also known as 'bruisewort' and is similar in its healing action to the better known Arnica (page 28). It is a cheerful and much loved plant with small, white petals and a sunny, yellow centre – a plant that nineteenth-century homoeopath John Henry Clarke describes as constantly being trodden on, only to bounce back up again. Culpeper, the seventeenth-century herbalist, used it widely for treating trauma, pleurisy, pneumonia and consumption of the lungs, and suggested that it grew in abundance because of its usefulness.

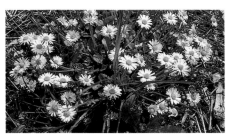

MAIN INDICATIONS

MENTAL AND EMOTIONAL

There is great exhaustion and a desire to lie down, although continual movement makes this patient feel better.

PHYSICAL

Bellis perennis is used for deep trauma, strains, sprains, blows, falls and bruising, the latter feeling more internal than external. Bellis perennis is particularly good for injury to deep tissue following surgery that has left the patient with post-operative pain. It can be very helpful after a violent blow to the breast. If swelling remains after the initial use of Arnica (page 28) then Bellis perennis will help reduce this. It is particularly indicated after a painful fall on the coccyx.

Pregnant women may find it useful if they are having problems walking due to strained abdominal muscles or painful bruising from the movement or kicking of the baby. It is also useful when the woman experiences bearing down, labour-like pains after delivery.

The action on the blood vessels makes it a useful remedy for varicose veins that feel bruised, squeezed and throbbing.

The stomach feels very heavy and can be extremely sensitive to being touched by clothing. Patients have a strong desire for vinegar and pickled foods, but this may cause vomiting of acids. It may also be affected if cold drinks are taken when the stomach feels hot.

A sudden chill from getting cold or wet when over-heated is a symptom peculiar to Bellis perennis. However, the remedy should not be taken late at night as it can cause sleeplessness.

Common Uses
- Injury • Bruising • Pregnancy

MODALITIES

Worse: *injury;
surgery; sprains;
heat; becoming
cold or wet when
hot*
Better: *motion*

Bryonia

Bryonia is a tall, herbaceous, perennial climber with berries the size of a pea that hang in groups. It is found creeping and crawling very slowly in damp, dark areas, as if hiding from view. It climbs high, using its long tendrils to cling to whatever it can find for support. There are many species of Bryonia to be found, but it is the root of the black-berried *Bryonia alba* that is used in homoeopathy.

The root is large and fleshy, exuding a foul-smelling, milky resin, which has a violent, purgative action if consumed. Another deadly poison, known in France as the 'Devil's turnip', Bryonia has been used extensively for medicinal purposes, but with caution, as just fifteen berries can kill a child.

FULL NAME
Bryonia alba
(Plant family: Cucurbitacae)

COMMON NAME
• White bryony

MAIN INDICATIONS

MENTAL AND EMOTIONAL

The Bryonia type often feels alone, insecure and vulnerable. Their insecurity stretches to fears about poverty and fear of the future, and their sense of vulnerability is increased by a vague mental stupor. When unwell they need to withdraw, otherwise they are irritable and unpleasant patients. Their insecurity is borne out by the strange delusion that they want to go home even if they are already there, and in social situations they often feel threatened.

PHYSICAL

Ailments come on slowly, and it is important that Bryonia patients slow down.

Any movement exacerbates the pain, and they need to lie quietly in a dark room, in contrast to the Rhus Tox picture (page 90) where motion helps. The pain in Bryonia is relieved by strong, firm pressure and the patient will often lie on the painful side.

Dryness is an important symptom, especially as it affects the mucous membranes. This makes Bryonia an excellent remedy for pleurisy, when dryness and movement from the cough cause sticking pains on inhalation. Stools are also dry, almost as if burned, causing extreme constipation. Heat causes aggravation, but drinking water and keeping cool bring great relief.

Common Uses
• Coughs • Bronchitis • Flu • Headaches
• Injuries • Constipation.

MODALITIES

Worse: *becoming hot; moving about; being touched; taking cold; lying on painless side; during sleep; in the morning*

Better: *warmth and pressure on the painful part; in cool, damp air; being quiet; being in a dark room; drawing up knees; applying cold water; eating cold foods; belching*

FULL NAME
Calcarea carbonica

SOURCE
• Oyster shell

Calc carb

This remedy is made from the soft inner layer of the oyster shell, which is lined with chalk and limestone. Oysters are molluscs that lie wide open on the sea bed, displaying their soft, snowy-white interiors. It takes just one, small disturbance for the shells to snap shut in an instant, showing a hard, impenetrable exterior. These elements are fundamental to the picture of Calc carb: the rock-like exterior covering the vulnerable interior.

Calcium is of vital importance to the body. It is the main component of bone, thereby providing us with our framework, and is the most widely present element in our bodies. It affects our metabolism and keeps sodium, potassium and magnesium in equilibrium. Without a sufficient balance of calcium we can easily become malnourished, stunting our development.

MAIN INDICATIONS

MENTAL AND EMOTIONAL

Calc carb is vitally important at times in our life when we need most stability and support. In the early stages of childhood, this remedy is useful for the solidity and strength that is needed for the future. It is thought that 40–50% of babies will need Calc carb.

This remedy can help us through puberty as we move into adulthood, and during old age it supports the movement away from the physical realm into one that is more spiritual.

Calc carb types tend to be quite happy, jolly people who know where they are, providing they have a secure home, enough money and a safe environment for themselves and their loved ones.

Work is important to Calc carb characters, who are generally highly industrious, with a great sense of responsibility. However, they will work only at their own pace, which is usually slow and methodical. Anything that threatens their much-loved security brings up many fears: fear of poverty, health, heights and even insanity. This last fear – that of insanity – is brought on by other fears, especially fear of the unknown and loss of control. Calc carb types are also anxious about others perceiving these fears, which leads them to object to being watched.

The exterior shell of the oyster is represented in a patient's ability to be incredibly stubborn and obstinate. Calc carbs are no-nonsense people who need to be met half-way, although they will ultimately do anything for anybody.

PHYSICAL

Calc carb babies tend to be flabby and unfit, rather like an oyster without the shell. They are slow to walk and talk, and their teething is often delayed and difficult. They can have unusually large heads that are sweaty, which, as with their feet, can smell sour. Their bellies are round and the fontanels are often late to close. There is a lot of mucus, and they can be prone to enlarged glands, although, in general, their constitution is quite strong. Constipation is common, but because this gives them more time it fits in well with the Calc carb picture and tends not to distress them; any stools are often pale, resembling chalk or clay. If the constipation changes to diarrhoea, however, patients become agitated.

The sourness in children is also present in adults. This is especially true in the alimentary canal, as diarrhoea and vomit will have a particularly unpleasant odour. Any exertion is difficult, and a tendency to be overweight causes them to perspire very easily. The bones are brittle and break easily, and osteoporosis can develop easily, due to the inability to absorb calcium.

There is a love of eggs, sugar, cakes, pastries and pasta, which only heightens their flabby nature. Calc carb people also have a strange desire for indigestible things, such as chalk.

Milk is something that they will either love or hate. They will be prone to sour vomiting, and Calc carb children will often vomit curdled milk, especially while teething.

Abscesses frequently occur, which are spongy, not hard, and uterine fibroids are quite common. The skin can often take a long time to heal after any injury. There is a convulsive tendency, and menstruation can be heavy – particularly around the time of the menopause – and involve painful cramping.

The musculo-skeletal system is greatly affected in the Calc carb patient, with rheumatism and arthritis commonplace. The pains usually start in the lower back and then gradually extend to other areas. Most of the skeletal problems are aggravated by cold, wet weather and eased by warmth.

Common Uses
- Teething • Ailments in children
- Backache

MODALITIES

Worse: *being cold; exercise and exertion; teething; puberty; milk; anxiety; after eating; sexual excesses*

Better: *dry weather; morning; passing wind; lying on their back; being in a dark room*

39

Calc fluor

FULL NAME
Calcarea fluorica

SOURCE
• Fluoride of lime

Calc fluor is an insoluble salt that is found naturally in the body, aiding the strength of the bone structure, teeth and tissue elasticity. It is one of twelve homoeopathic remedies, known as tissue salts, that are present in the tissues of the body.

MAIN INDICATIONS

MENTAL AND EMOTIONAL

In most of the Calc remedy types there is a need for security. In Calc fluor characters this is expressed by a fear of poverty. They tend to be quick-witted and grasp ideas easily but have an underlying chaotic tendency that can let them down. They can be clumsy and lack coordination.

PHYSICAL

As a tissue salt, the remedy Calc fluor is used to support various parts of the body that have lost tone and structure. It can also be used as a supplement, helping to strengthen teeth enamel. It also helps to soften areas of the body that have become hard, such as glands in the tonsils or neck, and redress bony growths, such as on the head or jaw line. Similarly, it is a good treatment for corns when the skin has become hard.

Lack of elasticity is a typical symptom of the Calc fluor patient, making it a useful prevention against stretch marks during pregnancy. Its affinity with the venous system means that it is also effective against chilblains – where the skin is badly cracked and chapped – improving the elasticity of the blood vessel walls and helping to improve circulation. It can be a good support remedy when there is a tendency towards varicose veins or haemorrhoids caused by a loss of tone in the walls of the blood vessels.

All discharges are thick and yellowy-green. Hence, Calc fluor can be useful for long-term catarrh, suppuration of the middle ear and adenoids.

Tendons and ligaments that have been strained may benefit from Calc fluor, especially if the injury is less severe when it is kept moving but feels worse for being rested. This is also applicable to other structural pains, such as in the lower back, making it similar to the remedy Rhus tox (page 90); in fact, Calc fluor can be used if Rhus Tox fails to help.

Common Uses
• Stretch marks • Varicose veins
• Chilblains • Haemorrhoids • Tooth decay
• Injuries

MODALITIES

Worse: *when starting to move; sprains and strains; cold and damp*
Better: *constant movement; warm applications; heat*

Calc phos

FULL NAME
Calcarea phosphorica

SOURCE
• Calcium phosphate

Adding phosphoric acid to lime water creates Calc phos. Within this remedy we see a combination of two of the most widely used remedies in the Materia Medica, Calc carb (page 38) and Phosphorus (page 84). Calc carb is a slow, steady remedy, and Phosphorus is fast and furious, so in Calc phos we see a combination of the two. Calcium carbonate and calcium phosphate are two of the most important constituents of bone, and this remedy has, therefore, a great affinity with the bones and the early formation of the skeleton.

MAIN INDICATIONS

MENTAL AND EMOTIONAL

This remedy is, perhaps, most useful in early childhood or during adolescence. Imagine stroppy, discontented children or teenagers who don't know what they want and can't articulate their problems, and a Calc phos image will begin to emerge. Calc phos types feel tired and sluggish and can't concentrate. They may dread going to school, which brings on anxiety and diarrhoea.

Many of these symptoms are exacerbated by malnutrition at a time when huge growth spurts are experienced. The flair and brightness are there, but the patients do not have the energy to express them. Stimulation from a social occasion helps to distract them from their malaise.

PHYSICAL

Lime is essential to bone growth and healthy teeth, and in this picture we find problems with late teething in a child, sometimes accompanied by green, spluttery diarrhoea. The teeth may be soft, with swollen, painful gums. The mouth tastes unpleasant, and the tongue may become blistered. The child may be intolerant of the mother's milk and vomit on feeding.

Assimilation of essential nutrients is a problem here. The bones can be brittle and soft, and curvature of the spine may occur. It also helps to knit fractured bones back together.

Calc phos is excellent during convalescence as it stimulates healthy cell division and digestion, stimulating the appetite. Calc phos patients, however, cannot bear to eat or drink cold things. Fresh air can also worsen the symptoms, especially headaches.

Common Uses
• Teething • Fractures • Exhaustion
• Promoting growth • Convalescence

MODALITIES

Worse: *changing seasons; teething; dampness; adolescence*
Better: *resting; warm weather*

Cantharis

FULL NAME
Cantharides

SOURCE
• Spanish fly
• Blister beetle

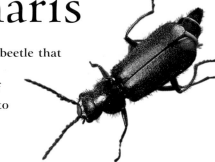

The Spanish fly is a small, green-blue beetle that excretes cantharidine, an irritant that produces an unpleasant blistering of the skin. The whole insect is ground to powder in the making of this remedy.

MAIN INDICATIONS

MENTAL AND EMOTIONAL

The irritant nature of the Spanish fly is reflected in the emotional picture of Cantharis types. They can have violent tempers that make them want to lash out at other people. They seem frenzied, and their language can be uncontrollably foul, containing sexual swear-words. There can be great sexual excitement and an erotic mania that isn't relieved by sex. Bright light or shiny objects can be aggravating to Cantharis types, and they can have a great fear of water. They can seem possessed and then suddenly lose consciousness or lapse into a stupor.

PHYSICAL

The sensation of burning dominates this remedy. Burning pain accompanies all the ailments suffered. The urinary tract is the most affected, and Cantharis is a soothing remedy for the unpleasant condition cystitis. Violent burning and cutting pains are felt in the bladder. There is a constant urge to urinate but it is only excreted little by little, causing spasms, scalding and pain; there may even be traces of blood. Overall, this is a particularly agonizing condition.

The throat also has a burning sensation, making swallowing difficult. There is an intense thirst, but the patient has a fear of drinking because it aggravates the pain. Even touching the larynx can send spasms through the body and cause breathing difficulties.

For burning conjunctivitis, Cantharis is a useful remedy to consider. The eyes are inflamed and they feel as if they are burning; tears feel as if they are scorching the face. The eyes can have a staring quality in a face that is hot and flushed.

Cantharis can also be used to help to heal burns that look raw, with smarting, stinging pains or when the skin is badly blistered.

MODALITIES

Worse: *looking at bright, shiny objects; drinking; touching the larynx; moving about*

Better: *being warm; resting; being quiet*

Common Uses
• Cystitis • Burns • Conjunctivitis
• Sore throats

Carbo veg

FULL NAME
Carbo vegetabilis

SOURCE
• Wood charcoal

Charcoal is familiar to most of us. Makers of this remedy originally took it from birch trees, but now it is prepared from beech wood.

The process by which charcoal is made gives an indication of how this remedy is best used. The wood is slowly heated until red hot, driving out the oxygen; then it is smothered in a closed container to carbonize, creating the compact but fragile substance. It is the slow eking out of the oxygen that corresponds so well to our picture of Carbo veg, with cyanosis and respiratory weakness presenting major problems in this remedy picture.

MAIN INDICATIONS

MENTAL AND EMOTIONAL

Carbo veg has often been referred to as the 'corpse reviver', presenting a picture of very low vitality, even stagnation. There is a definite lack of reaction on all levels. Emotionally, on a less acute level, there is a dull, exhausted indifference to life; patients are too tired to know how they really feel and don't seem to care if they are alive or dead. They do, however, have a strange fear of ghosts, and there is a marked anxiety and uneasiness in the dark.

PHYSICAL

The low vital signs lead to poor circulation, making patients feel very cold and clammy. Their skin is pale, with even a blue tinge due to lack of oxygen. In a situation of collapse or fainting they have a great need for air and are helped enormously by being fanned – the keynote of this remedy picture. Asthma attacks are common: the breathing is short and laboured so they need direct air into their lungs; an open window is a great relief, although cold air may bring on an attack. Circulation is poor, and varicose veins, which may ulcerate and blacken, are common.

The digestive symptoms of this remedy are also distinctive – charcoal tablets are still used for correcting acidity in the stomach. There is a great deal of bloating, especially in the upper abdomen, accompanied by excessive flatulence.

The Carbo veg patient feels exhausted, so this remedy is particularly useful when someone has had a debilitating illness from which they have never fully recovered.

Common Uses

• Flatulence • Indigestion • Asthma
• Coughs • Fainting

MODALITIES

Worse: *eating rich and fatty foods; being too warm; after debilitating illness; pressure of clothes around the waist; walking in fresh air*

Better: *being fanned; belching; passing wind; lying down*

Caulophyllum

FULL NAME
Caulophyllum thalictroides
(Plant family: Berberidaceae)

COMMON NAMES
- Blue cohosh
- Squaw root

Blue cohosh is found growing in the United States and Canada. It flourishes in damp, rich soils and flowers during May and June, displaying small yellow and green petals. The seeds can grow to the size of a pea and can be roasted to make a drink similar to coffee, although the taste is more bitter. The homoeopathic remedy is made from the root of the plant.

MAIN INDICATIONS

MENTAL AND EMOTIONAL

In Caulophyllum cases the patient feels extremely exhausted: this remedy is particularly useful in labour where the mother feels useless, tearful and unable to continue with the birthing process. There is fear and apprehension, and the memory is weakened. Caulophyllum types have mood swings, sometimes to the point of hysteria.

PHYSICAL

Caulopyllum is an invaluable remedy in childbirth when the labour pains are both short and very painful. The mother feels exhausted and there is rigidity of the cervix, which will not open. The afterpains are spasmodic, with cramping across the lower abdomen. Exhaustion prevents the uterus from cramping down properly to expel the placenta, therefore only partially expelling it or even retaining it. The lochia (discharge from the uterus after childbirth) may last an unusually long time or be totally absent as the womb is too inactive. The uterus feels very sore and the woman does not want to be touched.

The period pain of this remedy starts in the small of the back. The blood doesn't flow easily, and nausea, coupled with vomiting, can be a common occurrence. The pains are cramping, sharp and unpredictable. The symptoms are much better when the patient is warm, cold being felt easily. A strong thirst is also common.

Another feature of Caulophyllum is the tendency to joint pain. A lot of joints will crack and there may be severe drawing pains, which can fly about the body arbitrarily. The smaller joints tend to be more affected, such as the fingers and toes. The pain often leads to very restless nights.

MODALITIES

Worse: *during labour; in the evening*
Better: *warmth*

Common Uses
- Labour • Period pains • Rheumatism

Causticum

Causticum is a combination of calcium hydroxide, also known as marble, and potassium bisulphate, and was made and introduced by Samuel Hahnemann. Homoeopathically, it combines the traits of two groups of remedies, the Calcs and the Kalis, some of which are discussed in this book.

FULL NAME
Causticum

SOURCE
• Calcium hydroxide and potassium bisulphate

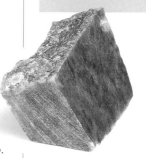

MAIN INDICATIONS

MENTAL AND EMOTIONAL

We find deeply sympathetic and sensitive people in this remedy. They generally start life with an open, lively character, which gradually gets battered by what life throws at them, leaving them emotionally paralysed. It is a useful remedy for grief, especially for those who suppress their emotions.

Causticum patients abhor injustice, but their stubborn stand against it often brings on mental and emotional paralysis. The mind begins to shut down: they forget where they have put things, and they can be prone to stuttering, especially if they are very excited or anxious. They are generally insecure: they don't like being alone, nor do they like the dark.

PHYSICAL

As well as mental paralysis there can also be physical paralysis, but usually only of specific parts. Ailments such as constipation or urinary incontinence, especially in the elderly, are common. Paralysis of the bladder can also occur after retention of urine or when the bladder has become too distended. Coughing, sneezing or laughing can cause the particular symptom of involuntarily urinating. Patients may also wet the bed on going to sleep.

Causticum is one of the great remedies for serious burns. It will help to relieve the raw, burning pains that are common in this picture as well as to heal scar tissue.

The cough in this picture is a deep, dry, hard and scraping one, hurting the chest. It is often brought on by cold, dry winds and is easily provoked by a tickle in the throat. It is very difficult to cough deeply enough always to dislodge the mucus. Small sips of water will ease the cough but lying in bed makes it much worse.

Warts are very common, especially on the hands, face and eyelids. Causticum types tend to be chilly but are worse for both heat and cold. In addition, they crave smoked food.

Common Uses
• Grief • Burns • Coughs

MODALITIES

Worse: *cold, dry winds; drafts; lying down; entering warm rooms after being in the cold*
Better: *warm air; warmth of the bed; damp weather*

Chamomilla

FULL NAME
Matricaria recutita
(Plant family: Compositae)

COMMON NAMES
• German camomile
• Wild camomile

Camomile is a European plant familiar to many, particularly as a herbal tea. It is related to the daisy and has similar flowers, which are just under 1 inch (20 mm) in diameter, with narrow white petals around a golden centre. It tends to flourish mainly in September, but may bloom earlier. These plants love sunshine and are rarely found in damp or shady areas, preferring roadsides and open cornfields. There is a certain untidiness to the plant, with straggly stems rising above the bushy and spindly, fern-like foliage. Camomile grows fairly rapidly, finishing its growing cycle within two months, and often providing a second crop.

There is an energy and exaggerated quality to the Chamomilla type, which is profiled below. The aroma is strong and slightly sweet yet, when tasted, there is a distinct bitterness. The essential oil is a deep blue colour and is said to be excellent for inflammation. In fact, there is a great deal of inflammation in the remedy picture of Chamomilla, especially on the emotional level.

MAIN INDICATIONS

MENTAL AND EMOTIONAL

Chamomilla types tend to have very short tempers. Their highly strung natures often give way to excessive irritability, where everything seems to make them angry. They are demanding, dissatisfied and generally very temperamental.

They have a very low pain threshold. Any pain they feel will be vocalized by screaming, shouting and even stamping about – not necessarily for attention, but to vent the agony they feel and hopefully purge the pain. Teething children usually show a typical Chamomilla picture. The pain in teething is obviously bad, but it often seems to them that little is being done to soothe their anguish. Very little calms teething children: toys, for example, are demanded, then thrown across room; they want to be held, perhaps rocked back and forth, but then scream as soon as this motion is stopped.

Chamomilla characters are so sensitive to pain and loathe it so much that they resent the illness and pain they are suffering and take out their anger and frustration on those around them. Such high emotions are felt in the stomach; how this effects the digestive system is described below in the physical profile. Stimulants such as coffee and narcotics have a profound effect on mood, heightening angry and aggressive behaviour.

Chamomilla will often help a woman in labour, where pain is almost unbearable. She may scream resentfully at her partner, cursing him for the pregnancy, even though he may be trying to help by holding her hand and trying to keep her calm and focused; Chamomilla types hate to be touched or spoken to when they are going through any kind of trauma.

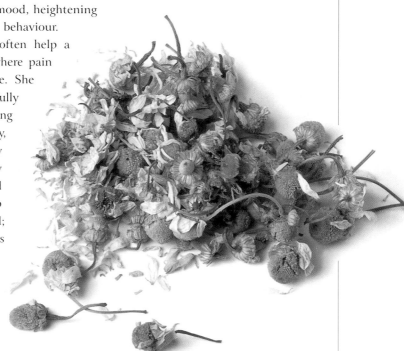

PHYSICAL

The teething child will feel a great need to be angry: the gums are swollen, tender and inflamed. One cheek will be red and hot, the other cool and pale. All heat makes the situation worse for them, particularly between 9 p.m. and midnight. Bouts of flatulence often accompany the teething problems, and diarrhoea may be present, which has the appearance and odour of chopped egg and spinach.

Chamomilla patients need to tuck themselves up and then extend their bodies to relieve colicky pain that makes them intensely restless. Colic can also be brought on by drinking too much coffee or after overindulging.

Chamomilla heads and feet can be particularly hot and sweaty, and restlessness can predominate sleep patterns. They will suffer with spells of jumpiness, jerking and twitching, which, once again, are much worse between 9 p.m. and midnight.

In Chamomilla, as with Pulsatilla (page 88), there may be acute earache, accompanied by anger, irritability and a flushed face. The pain may be exacerbated after exposure to cold.

Common Uses
• Teething • Earache • Diarrhoea
• Labour • Pain • Colic

MODALITIES

Worse: *teething; cold air; coffee; drugs; heat; late in the evening; drafts*

Better: *sweating; being carried; mild or warm, wet weather; cold applications*

China

FULL NAME
Cinchona officinalis
(Plant family: Rubiaceae)

COMMON NAMES
• Peruvian bark

The remedy China comes from the quinaquina tree, which grows at high altitude in the Andes of Peru and Ecuador. As well as growing alongside many other species, the tree can also be found growing alone as high as 9,000 feet (2,740 m). It stands tall and proud, the blossom exuding a delicate scent. There are many alkaloids contained in the bark, most famously quinine, which is still used extensively for the treatment of malaria.

This remedy was Hahnemann's first proving (page 9), and his discoveries after taking the bark in large quantities led him to develop homeopathy.

MAIN INDICATIONS

MENTAL AND EMOTIONAL

The world is a difficult place for China patients, who feel sensitive, debilitated and, like the tree on the mountainside, vulnerable. They are delicate and refined and need to be handled carefully – like bone china. The harsh reality of the outside world sometimes tempts China types to resort to a fantasy world.

PHYSICAL

The exhaustion and weakness felt by China types can be extreme, resulting mainly from a loss of fluids. China is a helpful tonic after childbirth if a lot of blood has been lost. It also helps during an intermittent fever when there is profuse sweating or following chronic bouts of diarrhoea that totally debilitate the patient. Of course, an intermittent fever, numbness, anxiety, a hard, small pulse and mental stupor make up the symptom picture for malaria, which the raw material of China – the bark – has long been administered as a cure.

There can be digestive disturbances with China. Flatulence and bloating are very common, but the symptoms are not relieved by passing wind or burping. Just as they cannot assimilate the world, China patients find food digestion very difficult: diarrhoea may contain undigested food. They have a craving for sweet and delicate food, but coarse foods, such as fats and bread, aggravate their digestive systems; fruit can often bring on diarrhoea. Everything they eat tastes salty and bitter.

China types are extremely sensitive, even to the lightest touch, although oddly, hard pressure eases their pain. Drafts and cold air tend to worsen things.

MODALITIES

Worse: *loss of fluids from anywhere in the body; cold winds; drafts; fruit*
Better: *hard pressure; bending double; fasting for a few days*

Common Uses

• Exhaustion • Bloating • Flatulence
• Diarrhoea • Malaria • Fever

Cocculus

Cocculus is found on the coast of Malabar in India and in Sri Lanka. It is a climbing plant, with yellow flowers and large, heart-shaped leaves on long stalks. It bears reddish-brown berries the size of a pea, which contain within them a poison called picrotoxin. Local fishermen used to throw the berries into the rivers to drug the fish. The fish would lose their ability to swim and eventually drown, as their gills filled with water, and the fishermen would gather the floating bodies. The picrotoxin poison has also been used in beer to make it seem stronger. The toxin does actually cause staggering and incoherent speech, familiar symptoms of someone who has had too much to drink.

FULL NAME
Anamirta cocculus
(Plant family:
Menispermaceae)

COMMON NAMES
• Indian cockle
• Fish berry

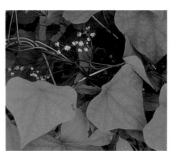

MAIN INDICATIONS

MENTAL AND EMOTIONAL

Cocculus types appear to be slightly disconnected: their speech is slow and they may find it difficult to understand what is being said to them. Slowness frequently alternates with wit and chattiness, however, which may bring on hysterics. They can seem weak and worn out and generally react in a dazed and confused fashion.

This is an excellent remedy if the patient is suffering from sleep deprivation, due to looking after other people. They are worn out and anxious from their duties. They can have a feeling that time passes too quickly. There may be a sense of sadness – many of the symptoms stem from grief.

PHYSICAL

Patients feel very nauseous and wobbly on their feet, often vertiginous, making

Cocculus one of the best remedies for travel sickness. Any motion will worsen the symptoms, even sitting down or standing up, or looking out of the window when travelling. The thought of food or drink will also make patients feel extremely sick, although they will generally feel thirsty. There may be flatulence and diarrhoea, distention of the stomach and griping pains. A bitter taste in the mouth and an increase in saliva may accompany burping.

A headache at the back of the head is another common feature of this remedy, also causing nausea. Any exposure to cold air will worsen the patient's condition.

Common Uses
• Travel sickness • Hangovers • Vertigo

MODALITIES

Worse: *moving to sit down or stand up; travelling by car; lack of sleep; noise; thought of food or drink; grief, anxiety*
Better: *resting; being still*

Coffea

FULL NAME

Coffea cruda

(Plant family: Rubiaceae)

COMMON NAME

• Unroasted coffee beans

Most of us are familiar with coffee and its stimulating effect, whether it is drunk first thing each morning to give a kick-start to the day, or late at night after a meal, frequently leaving us to toss and turn in search of sleep. Coffee is a stimulant that alerts the brain and acts on the central nervous system. If you have ever drunk several cups in a short time, this remedy picture is easy to understand.

MAIN INDICATIONS

MENTAL AND EMOTIONAL

Coffea does not allow the brain to switch off because the patient is stimulated both mentally and physically. As a result, it is one of the main remedies for insomnia, when thoughts race around the mind, preventing sleep. Brilliant ideas may spring to mind that are so exciting that sleep is impossible, or a dread from the day may linger in the mind. All the senses in this remedy feel more acute than normal: touch, smell and sounds are all heightened, possibly leading to feelings of agitation.

This is an excellent remedy for labour, when the mother feels sensitive to her surroundings. The sound of anyone talking, or even the smell of the room, becomes irritating. Pain can seem unbearable, and the patient may also suffer from an unshakeable fear of dying.

Incessant talking is a common feature of Coffea types, almost to the point of mild hysteria. They can be exceptionally funny and joyful, when the joy is so intense that it may cause crying or even palpitations.

PHYSICAL

Just as the mind is alert and sensitive, so the body reacts in the same way, feeling acutely sensitive to pain of any sort. The patient experiences extreme restlessness and is reluctant to be touched. They may feel too hot, suffer from palpitations or appear flushed, although they prefer not to be in the fresh air, as any exposure to cold only heightens their condition. Excessive emotion can cause painful headaches, which feel as if a nail is being driven into the side of the head.

Coffea is useful for toothache, when the nerve pain feels better for swilling cold water around the mouth.

Common Uses

• Insomnia • Hyperactivity • Toothache

MODALITIES

Worse: *cold air; noise; touch; over-excitement*

Better: *resting; ice-cold water*

50

Colocynth

FULL NAME

Citrullus colocynthis
(Plant family:
Cucurbitaceae)

COMMON NAME

• Bitter cucumber
• Bitter apple

Colocynth is a gourd belonging to the same family as Bryonia (page 37), trailing along the ground in a similar fashion. The fruit has a thin rind and looks similar to an orange. It is bitter in taste and was used as a purgative by ancient medics. If taken in large quantities, vomiting and nausea can become so intense that death may result. The homoeopathic remedy is made from the fruit once it has been dried and reduced to a powder.

MAIN INDICATIONS

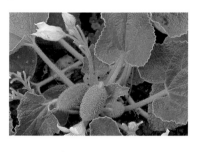

MENTAL AND EMOTIONAL.

Many of the symptoms that we find in this remedy are brought on by emotional states. Colocynth types are easily offended, and emotions such as anger or humiliation will cause the cramping and agitated state that we see on the physical level. They don't want to see or talk to anyone, preferring to hide their distressed state. Their pain may become so intense, however, that they cry out loud in agony. Children are angry and restless and may scream if they are picked up.

PHYSICAL

Pain is extremely violent, with cramping, twisting, gnawing and pinching sensations. Relief comes from heat and very hard pressure, such as a fist being pushed into the abdomen, or bending over double. Lying on the abdomen or on the affected part can also help.

Many of the symptoms occur around the stomach, abdomen and ovaries, and, as such, Colocynth is a useful remedy for food poisoning. Nausea will accompany the cramping, colicky pains and patients will vomit until the stomach is empty. Any diarrhoea is usually white and ropy.

Pain will often come in waves, leaving the patient exhausted and unable to speak. Menstrual cramps can be relieved by Colocynth, together with hard pressure on the abdomen and warmth. This remedy also eases neuralgia, and is helpful for sciatica, when there are shooting pains that feel better when lying on the affected side.

It is important to examine the causation carefully before administering this remedy, however, as many symptoms will come from an emotional situation, long-term anxiety, irritability or anger.

Common Uses

• Colic • Diarrhoea • Gastroenteritis
• Period pains

MODALITIES

Worse: *emotion, such as anger or irritation; being offended; during the evening*

Better: *heat; hard pressure; bending double; lying on the abdomen*

Drosera

FULL NAME
Drosera rotundifolia
(Plant family:
Droseraceae)

COMMON NAME
• Sundew

Drosera grows close to the ground in the wet, boggy highlands of Scotland, among the heather. It has cup-shaped leaves, which grow on stumpy stalks. Each leaf has red hairs, exuding a sticky substance that glistens in the sunlight, hence its name 'sundew'. Although delightful in appearance, these hairs are used to trap unsuspecting insects, which are then devoured by this carnivorous plant.

MAIN INDICATIONS

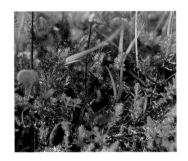

MENTAL AND EMOTIONAL

Drosera patients are irritated by the slightest criticism. Their obstinacy is infuriating as they insist on carrying out their ideas, despite the objections of others. They can also feel restless and find it difficult to concentrate on anything for longer than a few minutes, before getting bored and moving on to the next task.

The Drosera type can easily become anxious and paranoid, doubting the motives of others. On the other hand, they cannot bear to be alone, especially if they wake up in the middle of the night when they are ill. They may even fear ghosts.

PHYSICAL

The cough in the Drosera picture is the most predominant feature, and this can, therefore, be an excellent remedy for whooping cough. Patients feel suffocated by the cough because it comes in fits, making breathing difficult. The cough sounds deep, hollow and barking, and sufferers may feel that they have to hold the sides of their chest to support themselves. In addition, patients can cough up bitter-tasting, yellow sputum, and the severity of the cough can even rupture blood vessels, causing nosebleeds. Patients' suffering is much worse for lying down, and, therefore, worse at night when going to sleep. Heat also aggravates the symptoms, with fresh air and moving about soothing the pain. The tickling sensation that occurs in the throat inevitably brings on another coughing fit, and the voice generally becomes hoarse, so that talking or laughing also prompt coughing.

The face may look flushed and hot but the rest of the body will feel cold, with cold sweating during the night. The patient feels weak, and their eyes may be sunken.

Common Uses
• Coughs • Asthma

MODALITIES

Worse: *heat; lying down; at night; talking; laughing*
Better: *moving around; cool, fresh air; sitting up*

Eupatorium

Boneset is a perennial herb that grows in damp meadows. It was used by the North American Indians for colds and flu and is still used extensively today in herbal medicine.

FULL NAME
*Eupatorium
perfoliatum*
(Plant family:
Compositae)

COMMON NAME
• Boneset

MAIN INDICATIONS

MENTAL AND EMOTIONAL

The patient feels exhausted and, as a result, capable of very little, except, perhaps, moaning and crying from the pain.

PHYSICAL

There is a great deal of restlessness and pain in this remedy picture.

Eupatorium is excellent for colds, flu and fevers, especially when the bones feel incredibly painful, as if they are broken. During flu, the pain is felt deep inside the bone with an intense aching and a sensation of being bruised all over. Chills start in the small of the back, causing the patient to shudder and perhaps sweat, but only mildly. Sweating, however, often seems to relieve the symptoms.

There is a desperate desire to be as warm as possible, although once warm patients may feel as if they are burning up. Catarrh can often be copious, and there may be a constant urge to sneeze.

Eupatorium types would much rather simply lie down and sleep until they feel better, but the restlessness and pain make it impossible for them to do so. Headaches throb in the brain and, unlike flu, feel worse with any sweating. The eyeballs ache and feel extremely tender.

Any thought of food can often make Eupatorium patients feel sick, although they crave water, despite the fact that it often makes the symptoms much worse. Having felt worse for drinking water, however, they frequently become frightened to drink.

Common Uses
• Colds • Flu • Fever

MODALITIES

Worse: *being cold; staying still; the thought of food; drinking water*
Better: *sweating*

Euphrasia

FULL NAME
Euphrasia officinalis
(Plant family: Scrophulariaceae)

COMMON NAME
• Eyebright

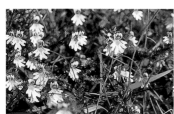

Euphrasia grows abundantly in Europe and North America in mountainous meadows and on high, chalky downs. The flowers are borne in upright racemes, and they are white with flecks of purple and yellow. Some say that, on close examination, it also resembles a bloodshot eye, a description that may have led to its first medicinal use. It has been used for many centuries; Milton describes in *Paradise Lost* how the Archangel Michael used this herb to enhance Adam's vision in the Garden of Eden.

The name Euphrasia comes from the Greek word meaning gladness, as it was thought that by restoring sight it gave joy to life.

MAIN INDICATIONS

MENTAL AND EMOTIONAL

There are no distinctive mental or emotional indications to note with this remedy.

PHYSICAL

It is logical that, with eyebright as a common name, Euphrasia is used to ease a multitude of eye problems. Any catarrhal condition of the eyes when the tears are acrid and burning is relieved by this remedy. These symptoms may appear together with a nose that is constantly runny during the day but gets stuffed up at night when the patient lies down. Euphrasia is also an excellent treatment for conjunctivitis or hay fever.

The eyelids can be sore, inflamed and very itchy, possibly oozing acrid pus; the eyeballs may appear bloodshot. On waking, the eyes may be stuck together and be difficult to open. Euphrasia will help if the cornea has blistered and eyesight seems misty and blurred. The eyes may feel painful, gritty and sandy, and there may be intolerance to bright lights.

Euphrasia may also help to ease colds, although only when the cold generally moves down to the chest, causing coughing that is worse during the day but almost disappears at night when the sufferer lies down.

Patients will feel extremely chilly and find it difficult to warm up, although they will feel better for fresh air. They may also possibly show signs of fever.

Two drops of the Euphrasia tincture in some boiled, cooled water is excellent for external applications to the eyes.

Common Uses
• Conjunctivitis • Colds • Hay fever
• Eye injuries

MODALITIES

Worse: *bright light; being inside in a stuffy room; at night, for a runny nose; daytime, for a cough; windy weather*

Better: *fresh air; darkness*

Ferrum phos

White phosphate of iron is a tissue salt. It forms part of the haemoglobin in our red blood cells, carrying oxygen to all parts of the body and helping to strengthen veins and arteries. Ferrum phos is an extremely useful remedy in the first stages of illness, before any discharges have occurred. It is particularly good in treating anaemia, inflammation and fever.

FULL NAME
Ferrum phosphoricum

COMMON NAME
• White phosphate of iron

MAIN INDICATIONS

MENTAL AND EMOTIONAL

Ferrum phos patients are talkative, excitable and over-sensitive. They have mood swings and memory lapses, where forgetfulness is accompanied by anxiety about the future. Sadness, listlessness and depression displace courage and hope.

PHYSICAL

The patient feels much better for sleep. This is the remedy to use when the top of the head feels dull and heavy, with pain on one side, as if a nail is being driven in. Hammering pains are worse on the right side and feel better after a nosebleed or cold pressure. Ferrum phos is useful for children's headaches, especially when the eyes and face are red. Eyes are generally red and inflamed, with a burning sensation, as if a piece of grit is under the eyelid.

Ferrum phos can be effective in the early stages of an ear infection, when the symptoms include inflamed ears, radiating pains and pulsating, chronic catarrh of the middle ear.

This is also a good remedy for the initial stages of all inflammatory respiratory conditions, such as bronchitis, painful tickly coughs or croup, as well as loss of voice through hoarseness. Those who are susceptible to colds would do well to take Ferrum phos at the onset of any symptoms, especially a sore and ulcerated throat. The mucous membranes are congested in a similar way to the Aconite picture (page 20). Patients suffering from fevers when the face is flushed and the skin is hot and dry may also find Ferrum phos helpful.

Ferrum phos is a good remedy for both haemorrhoids and haemorrhaging, especially where the blood is bright red. For instance, it eases nosebleeds, and very heavy periods. It is used in combination with Calc phos (page 41) for cases of anaemia.

Common Uses
• Onset of a cold • Fever • Inflammation
• Nosebleeds • Anaemia • Earache

MODALITIES
Worse: *at night; moving about; noise*
Better: *having a nosebleed; slowing down; solitude*

55

FULL NAME
Gelsemium
sempervirens
(Plant family:
Loganiaceae)

COMMON NAME
• Yellow jasmine

Gelsemium

Gelsemium is a wonderfully scented climbing plant, displaying a magnificent set of bright yellow flowers, which bloom between March and May. It is found mainly in wooded areas and along the coastlines of the southern states of the United States. It flourishes in rich soils where its roots embed themselves deep into the ground for extra strength and support. As it climbs high, Gelsemium needs to fasten on to things around it. Although beautifully scented, it is a poisonous plant that, if consumed in its natural state, can cause paralysis and breathing difficulties. The root and stems are used in the preparation of the homoeopathic remedy.

MAIN INDICATIONS

MENTAL AND EMOTIONAL

In this remedy we find a picture of weakness, debility and paralysis, with an inability to hold oneself up. Gelsemium characters may experience anticipatory anxiety, with a dread of what is to come. Exams, interviews, public speaking or any new, previously unexperienced situations will all make them fearful. They may feel their legs giving way and shake with fear.

There is an element of cowardliness: Gelsemium types are much more inclined to admit defeat and withdraw than be confrontational. As a reaction, the mind has a difficulty in functioning properly, perhaps feeling paralysed. There is a heaviness in the head giving way to a feeling of dullness, stupidity and disconnectedness. Fear renders them speechless.

Initially, Gelsemium types may feel hysterical, as well as exhilarated and clear-headed, but this soon turns into a sense of heaviness and weakness. They can experience a great fear of heights, especially when landing in an aeroplane. This fear of downward motion is most clearly displayed by young children and babies, who scream as they are put in their cot.

Gelsemium is useful during labour if the contractions cease because the mother feels too scared to give birth.

PHYSICAL

Gelsemium is the main remedy used to treat heavy colds and flu. The classic symptoms of flu give an excellent insight into the Gelsemium picture. The condition starts slowly, making patients realize that they are are on the verge of illness. They feel exhausted and weak, and the throat feels sore. Chills and shivers run up and down the spine, and the legs feel heavy.

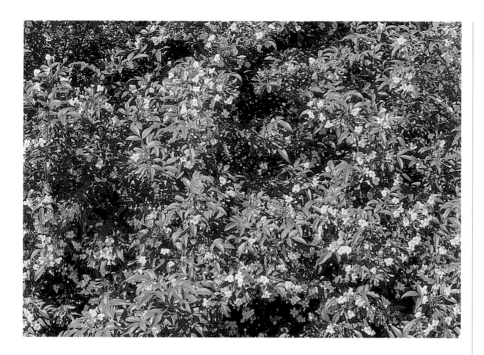

Gelsemium types can hardly move, as if their bodies are paralysed and numb. The eyelids feel extremely heavy, blurring the vision and making it difficult to focus. This condition has been likened to being in a glass coffin: the messages from the brain to the body do not get through. The patient is aware of what is going on but is unable to respond.

These flu-like symptoms may be accompanied by throbbing headaches that start at the back of the head, bringing tension to the neck and shoulders. The pain creeps forwards to the eyes and around the temples, or even the head, as if it is being held in a tight clasp. Thought and vision are foggy. Urinating can substantially alleviate the symptoms, especially the headaches and tension around the eyes. Alcohol also relieves the pain – partly by inducing urination.

Gelsemium is also a helpful remedy to administer to someone who has never fully recovered from flu. Patients can appear very over-heated, with a red, puffy face.

In a frightening situation, the body of the Gelsemium type can shut down and seem paralysed, possibly muting the patient temporarily. Anticipatory anxiety can bring on diarrhoea, which, although sometimes involuntary, is rarely painful. Heat and humidity tend to aggravate any symptoms.

Common Uses

• Flu • Colds • Fear • Shock

MODALITIES

Worse: *damp, humid environments; fear and shock; new situations*
Better: *urinating; alcohol; being in the open air*

Graphites

FULL NAME
Graphite

SOURCE
• Plumbago carbon

MODALITIES

Worse: *being cold; exercise; decision-making*

Better: *crying; talking to someone; being wrapped up; eating*

Graphite is a mineral carbon that contains no oxygen or hydrogen – the life has been burned out of it. This state is reflected in the emotional picture of this remedy. Incidentally, Graphites is made from the same carbon used for the lead in pencils.

MAIN INDICATIONS

MENTAL AND EMOTIONAL

The Graphites character is slow, sluggish and slightly apathetic. Patients lack confidence about life and struggle with their responses to certain situations. There is a great deal of confusion, slowness of memory and an overall uncertainty. With the doubts come anxiety and despair, and patients will ponder questions for hours but never arrive at a solution. Moods can fluctuate between anger, sadness and excitability.

Graphites types often work hard in a methodical fashion, making them seem uncomplicated on the surface – a thick skin, however, hides their inner sensitivity. Their condition improves after expressing their emotions by crying or talking through their problems, giving them a better idea of their priorities.

PHYSICAL

There is a tendency to be overweight in an unhealthy, rather unrobust way, or problems of malnutrition may be present. The skin symptoms are the most prominent: Graphites is a superb remedy for hard, cracked or crusty skin, especially, for example, in folds behind the ear or on the elbow. The skin can ooze either a clear, honey-like discharge or something resembling yellow glue. Cracks and fissures may form around the nose, eyes, mouth and anus, and the nails are misshapen and overly thick. Graphites can also be useful for treating scars if the old wound is lumpy, thick and hard, with a tendency to reopen.

Patients have a problem with elimination and may find it hard to sweat, although when they do it is unpleasant and staining. Constipation is common: the stools are large and knotty and may be held together with stringy mucus.

Graphites types feel cold most of the time yet like to be in fresh air if they are wrapped up warmly. There is a constant urge to eat, and they feel much better for doing so; warm milk gives great comfort.

Common Uses
• Eczema • Impetigo

58

Hamamelis

FULL NAME
Hamamelis
virginiana
(Plant family:
Hamamelidaceae)

COMMON NAME
• Witch hazel

Hamamelis looks like an apple tree and grows 10–12 feet (3–3.5 m) in height. Its flowers are yellow and grow in clusters, but they do not appear until late autumn. It has become a familiar household remedy due to its healing properties for burns and bruises, and was used historically by the North American Indians as a poultice for swellings.

MAIN INDICATIONS

MENTAL AND EMOTIONAL

Hamamelis patients are generally tired and weary, unable to communicate or do any work.

PHYSICAL

Hamamelis is mainly associated with treating haemorrhages, which may occur anywhere on the body. It can also be used to heal bruising, haemorrhoids and varicose veins.

The haemorrhoids are blue in colour, protruding and may bleed profusely. They are extremely sore and raw, and the rectum feels tremendously weighed down, so much so that it may feel as if the weight is too much to bear and will break the back. The pain is felt as a hot, burning sensation, and the haemorrhoids are very itchy.

With the hamamelis picture, all the veins feel swollen, inflamed and sore, as if bruised, and they are especially sore when touched. Varicose veins look knotted and feel hard, full and painful; they may possibly become ulcerated and bleed. Any bleeding will be helped by this remedy.

Hamamelis is also effective in the treatment of bloodshot eyes, especially when caused by violent coughing, or for black eyes when Arnica (page 28) has helped with the bruising but the eyesight is still hazy. The loss of blood can make the patient feel very tired.

Hamamelis will help to relieve most nosebleeds, especially those that continue for a long time or when the bridge of the nose feels quite tight.

Common Uses
• Haemorrhoids • Varicose veins
• Haemorrhages

MODALITIES

Worse: *pressure and touch; injuries; surgery; moving about*
Better: *resting and being still*

59

Hepar sulph

FULL NAME
Hepar sulphuris

SOURCE
• Calcium sulphide

Hepar sulph is an interesting remedy in that it is made from two quite opposing substances, calcium and sulphur, which are both homoeopathic remedies in their own right. Hepar sulph is made from equal parts of finely powdered oyster shells, Calc carb (page 38), and pure Sulphur (page 98), creating an explosive combination as it brings together the vulnerability of calcium and the fiery elements of sulphur.

MAIN INDICATIONS

MENTAL AND EMOTIONAL

This remedy picture reflects the highly vulnerable condition of the nervous system. Hepar sulph types tend to be very irritable, obstinate and malicious – all symptoms of their intolerance of external pressures and stresses. They can also be aggressive and argumentative.

Great anxiety, insecurity and fear are part of this picture, especially fear of darkness, both at night and on waking. Patients can also have a strange delusion that the world is on fire, as well as having pyromaniac tendencies.

PHYSICAL

Hepar sulph patients are extremely chilly. They cannot bear to touch anything cold, and the slightest draft will affect them. They love warmth and being in bed, however, and also feel better in more humid surroundings. This remedy is often used for colds that have dragged on and on, if Aconite (page 20) has already been tried.

Pains feel unbearable and are usually stitching, splinter-like pains, especially in the throat. The tonsils can be acutely inflamed, with pain extending up to the ears with every swallow or yawn. Hepar sulph is one of the main remedies used for tooth abscesses where pus is forming and the area feels very sore and tender.

There is a great deal of suppuration in this remedy, with thick, yellow, foul discharges. The cough is dry and croupy, with rattling in the chest and an inability to expel any mucus. It is much worse in the morning, and exposure to cold, dry winds may be the triggering mechanism. The skin is unhealthy with boils, carbuncles and abscesses oozing the same thick, yellow discharge.

A useful indication of this remedy is that patients will often crave acidic foods such as vinegar and pickles.

MODALITIES

Worse: *being cold; dry weather; uncovering; touch; noise; lying on the painful part; night-time*

Better: *warmth; damp weather*

Common Uses

• Abscesses • Boils • Coughs • Croup

Hypericum

FULL NAME
*Hypericum
perfoliatum*
(Plant family:
Clusiaceae)

COMMON NAME
• St John's wort

Hypericum is a rambling garden plant that produces vibrant yellow flowers. If you crush the flowers between your fingers they give off a rich, red juice that looks like blood – perhaps an indication to early herbalists of its medicinal uses as a wound healer.

Another particular feature of this plant is that the deep green leaves have small holes, which can be seen only when held up to sunlight. For a remedy that is commonly used for puncture wounds, these seem highly appropriate!

MAIN INDICATIONS

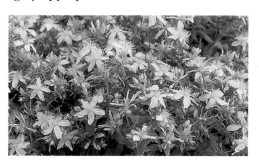

MENTAL AND EMOTIONAL

As a herbal remedy, Hypericum is well known in treating depression. Homoeopathically we find it useful in the treatment of depression after an injury or surgery. As with the remedy Arnica (page 28), the patient displays signs of shock, characterized by amnesiac tendencies and confusion, particularly after a head injury. Peculiarly, they can feel as if they are high in the sky, perhaps instilling a fear of heights.

PHYSICAL

Hypericum is another valuable first-aid remedy, known as the 'Arnica of the nerves' because it helps to ease the immense pain felt when parts of the body rich in nerves are injured. Crushed fingers, stubbed toes and spinal injuries – especially to the coccyx – are all helped by taking Hypericum. It is strongly indicated when the pain shoots upwards from the point of injury, and is stitching, darting or tearing in nature. This makes it a useful remedy whenever there is a possibility of tetanus.

Puncture wounds and lacerations from things such as surgical incisions and rusty nails, as well as head injuries which give way to convulsions due to violent, shooting pains, are also remedied by Hypericum. The wound will often be very inflamed and more painful than it looks.

Hypericum is known as a great antiseptic in tincture form. It can be applied to cuts, grazes and insect bites, and is often found in combination with Calendula (see table in Introduction – page 14).

Common Uses

• Injury to the nerves • Lacerated wounds
• Insect bites • Antiseptic

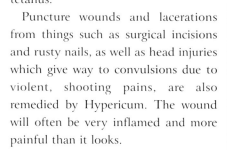

MODALITIES

Worse: *injury,
especially to the
nerves; touch;
puncture wounds;
lacerated wounds;
movement; damp
weather*
Better: *not moving;
bending the head
backwards*

61

Ignatia

FULL NAME
Strychnos ignatii or
Ignatia amara
(Plant family
Loganiaceae)

COMMON NAME
• St Ignatius's bean

St Ignatius's bean is the fruit from *Strychnos ignatii*, a beautiful plant found growing in Vietnam, China and the Philippines. It is a tall, woody, climbing shrub, which displays an array of tubular flowers, smelling of jasmine. These flowers bear a fruit about the size of a pear, containing around 24 seeds in the fleshy pulp. In the past, the seeds were worn around the neck as an amulet to guard against poisonous substances. Nowadays, however, the poisonous content of the seeds is used to make a powerful homoeopathic remedy.

Like the remedy Nux vomica (page 80), the seeds of the fruit are bitter and contain a high level of the poison strychnine, which makes up about 60% of the alkaloids. The poison affects the central nervous system: the respiratory centre is affected first, followed by muscular spasms and mental breakdown, leading to exhaustion and paralysis.

MAIN INDICATIONS

MENTAL AND EMOTIONAL

The general symptoms of Ignatia are the result of its traumatic emotional picture, which revolve around the themes of separation and loss. Events such as bereavement, miscarriage or the break up of a relationship are examples of such emotional upheaval.

In the acute situation that follows such a trauma, patients experience an emotional seizure: they neither believe nor understand what is happening to them. They can have difficulty in speaking, and what they do say is often incoherent. Some find it difficult to show emotion physically, even though it feels as if the emotion is stuck in their throat and they must constantly swallow to unblock it. They feel it is safer to suffer in silence. Others sob uncontrollably, sometimes suffering from bouts of hysteria with such violent movement that it would appear they were having an epileptic fit.

Another part of the Ignatia picture concerns mental conflict, especially with regard to the intelligent, romantic, capable patients. Ignatia types can be great idealists, expressing beliefs that conflict with what is socially acceptable. However, rather than stick to their ideals, they force themselves to go the way of the majority, suppressing their feelings, heightening the conflict inside.

Ignatia patients are often very capable people, but they can be rather scornful of those who are not. They may often be quick-witted, incisive, perceptive people, as well as deeply romantic. Although they may perceive the harsh realities of the world, their weak communication skills mean they tend to take on too much and end up burned-out wrecks. They are the type to put up a front in public and suffer in private.

Ignatia people are often difficult to live with. They can be moody and contradictory and, despite their awareness of their inclination to act as prima donnas, they continue to do so. This only makes matters worse by bringing on feelings of guilt and disappointment.

PHYSICAL

There is a strong tendency for the Ignatia type to have dramatic physical symptoms. The whole body physically cramps up: the stomach feels knotted and the chest in general feels compressed, making it very difficult to breathe. In order to get air into their lungs, Ignatia types must sigh or yawn heavily. They feel asthmatic, but it is better diagnosed as hysterical breathing.

Female patients' menses may be suppressed after a trauma. These patients too will give out long sighs and yawn frequently.

Frequent spasms, twitching, cramping and trembling, which can be either localized or spread over a large area of the body, are indicative of Ignatia. Also symptomatic is the inability to stop a coughing fit once started – patients have to be shocked out of it.

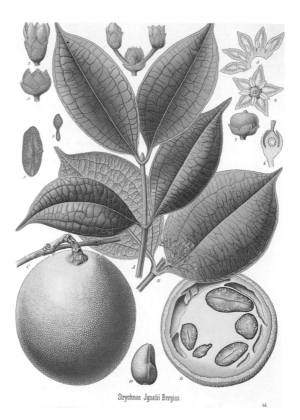

Strychnos Ignatii Bergius.

In an attempt to cope with their stress, the Ignatia type will often eat copiously, putting on large amounts of weight. Swallowing food seems to help ease the lump they often feel in their throats. They have an aversion to some foods, however, particularly fruit, and they loathe tobacco smoke.

As with Sepia (page 92), many of the symptoms of Ignatia may be relieved by physical exercise, such as walking very fast.

Common Uses
• Grief • Depression • Anxiety • Shock

MODALITIES

Worse: *emotion; consolation; touch; strong smells; coffee; tobacco; winter; mid-morning*
Better: *profuse urination; solitude; warmth; swallowing; hard pressure*

Ipecac

FULL NAME
Psychotria ipecacuanha
(Plant family: Rubiaceae)

COMMON NAME
• Ipecacuanha

Ipecac is a low-growing shrub that thrives in damp, shady areas in parts of Central and South America. The root of the plant, used to make the homoeopathic remedy, has been widely used over the centuries to treat diarrhoea and dysentery. More recently, it has been administered as an expectorant for catarrhal problems and asthma. The orthodox treatment was almost homoeopathic in its application because large quantities of the plant were known to cause considerable respiratory and digestive distress.

MAIN INDICATIONS

MENTAL AND EMOTIONAL

Ipecac patients are known for their ugly moods. They can be irritable and sulky and generally very difficult to satisfy. They rarely have much to say and can appear clumsy and awkward. Bottling up their emotions, however, may often trigger the symptoms.

PHYSICAL

Nausea is one of the most distinctive symptoms in the Ipecac picture; it seems to be present with nearly every complaint. Patients constantly have the urge to vomit but vomiting doesn't, unfortunately, alleviate the symptoms. The sight or smell of food only increases the urge, but the tongue looks clean and uncoated, in spite of the vomiting. However, considering the nausea, the lack of thirst in the Ipecac picture is perhaps surprising. The stools can be green and fermented, and there may also be some mucus and blood present.

The respiratory centre is also greatly affected. The patient feels suffocated by the coughing and vomiting, often making the face red or even blue because of the lack of air in the lungs. Any coughs are wheezing and rattling, and sound as if the lungs are full of mucus. This is similar to the remedy Ant Tart (page 23), with the difference that the Ipecac patient's symptoms will come on quite suddenly and vomiting generally brings up the mucus.

In an asthma attack or coughing fit there is a need to sit upright, and patients may want to stand next to an open window until breathing gets easier. They usually feel very chilly, and the body may become stiff and rigid.

MODALITIES

Worse: *warmth; over-eating; movement*
Better: *fresh air*

Common Uses
• Morning sickness • Nausea • Diarrhoea
• Cough • Bronchitis

64

Kali bich

Kali bich is made from the chromium of iron ore. It is highly poisonous if ingested, severely irritating the mucous membranes. It is used as a dye for material and wood.

FULL NAME
Kali bichromicum

SOURCE
• Bichromate of potash

MAIN INDICATIONS

MENTAL AND EMOTIONAL

The Kali bich character enjoys a world full of rules and regulations, where everything has to be done by the book. Patients need to know exactly where they stand, finding it hard to look beyond their own world or to be flexible. They are conscientious and like to be valued for their high standard of work.

PHYSICAL

Catarrhal problems are symptomatic in the Kali bich picture, especially in the upper nasal passages. Patients are frequently afflicted by colds, often leading to sinusitis. They have copious amounts of stringy, gluey catarrh that is white or yellow when there is an infection. Sometimes it is lumpy or comes out in huge globules – Kali bich is a great remedy for breaking up thick discharges.

The pain, which tends to come and go quite suddenly, lies at the bridge of the nose and can be pinpointed with the finger; pressure on this spot may give relief.

Patients may suffer from migraines or bad headaches, starting with blurred vision, which eases as time goes by. Again, the pain can be pinpointed at the pressure points. Vomiting mucus may relieve the headache. Light and noise aggravate the symptoms, as does stooping forward, but lying still in a darkened room helps to ease them.

Asthma attacks are common – they generally occur between 2 and 5 in the morning – during which time sitting up is imperative, and bending forwards, resting the head on the arms, helps a lot. Symptoms can vary, however. For example, rheumatic pains may appear once the catarrhal symptoms have disappeared, when the joints tend to be red and swollen. Alternatively, rheumatic pains may be followed by digestive symptoms, and so on.

Patients are chilly and dislike cold, although symptoms are often initially brought on by a change to warmer weather. There may be a desire for beer.

Common Uses
• Sinusitis • Catarrh • Asthma

MODALITIES

Worse: *being cold; warm or wet weather; 2–5 a.m.*
Better: *warm applications; vomiting mucus; lying still*

65

FULL NAME
Kali carbonicum

SOURCE
• Potassium
  carbonate

Kali carb

Kali carb is made from the ashes of vegetables, and it is mainly found in the earth and in plants. Within our own bodies potassium is a vital component of the cell structure.

MAIN INDICATIONS

MENTAL AND EMOTIONAL

We find a controlled, yet slightly dogmatic and materialistic, person in this remedy. Kali carb types are straightforward and don't tend to yield to emotion. They also operate on the basis of certainties: black is black and white is white. The fear of being alone leaves them desperate for company, and they can display signs of possessiveness. They tend to treat others rather badly, however, and do not like to be touched. Fears about health, the future and death are not suppressed by sleep, causing patients to wake between 2 and 5 in the morning in an agitated state because they feel out of control.

PHYSICAL

Kali carb characters are weak and worn down after many years of suppressed emotion. They tend to look pale and waxy and have puffy eyes; they also retain water very easily. This retention often causes painful lower back problems, as if everything gets stuck there, and the physical and emotional levels reflect one another. This is also true of digestive disorders, such as bloating and flatulence.

Kali carb is a good remedy during childbirth if the labour is delayed because the backache is too painful. All pains tend to be shooting, burning or tearing.

Patients always feel cold, and drafts irritate them intensely. They can catch cold easily, often made worse by their cold sweats. They produce thick, yellow catarrh, which often becomes crusty by the time they wake up in the morning.

Kali carb is also helpful for bronchitis, if the cough is dry and hacking in cold weather but loosens in the warmth. This can bring on asthma attacks, usually between 2 and 5 a.m., causing patients to wake fearfully, needing to put their elbows on their knees.

Common Uses
• Bronchitis • Asthma • Backache

MODALITIES

Worse: *being cold;*
  cold drafts
Better: *being warm*

Kali phos

Kali phos is one of the twelve homoeopathic remedies known as tissue salts, which are present in the tissues of the body.

FULL NAME
Kali phosphoricum

SOURCE
• Phosphate of potassium

MAIN INDICATIONS

MENTAL AND EMOTIONAL

Kali phos is an excellent remedy for nervous exhaustion. Patients are weak and weary, and their nerves feel on edge. They are nervous, anxious and find sleeping difficult. They may seem nervous and shy in company, with a tendency to blush easily. Their exhaustion can make them irritable and snappy, especially with the people they know and love, rather like the symptoms associated with the remedy Sepia (page 92).

PHYSICAL

Kali phos is a nerve nutrient and is excellent for muscular weakness and physical exhaustion. There is a lot of nervous tension, either from working too hard, over-excitement or prolonged worry. It is a good remedy for brain fatigue and may help cure a nervous headache – one that has been brought on by continued, intensive study, for example. It will help with insomnia when it is caused by nervous tension or being over-tired, such as in the case of jet lag.

Kali phos patients may suffer from nausea due to feeling nervous and will

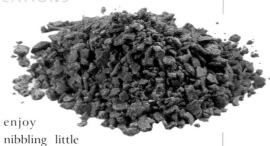

enjoy nibbling little bits of food to ease the sensation of emptiness felt in the stomach. The nerve-endings are affected, causing shooting pains throughout the patient's nervous system.

This remedy is an excellent tonic for shingles after the initial attack, as its capacity as a nerve nutrient helps to restore the nerves. Kali phos can also help counteract any nagging, dull toothache in teeth with fillings or which are decaying.

Most of the discharges in this picture will be yellow, including urine and stools, and are likely to smell foetid. Patients can often have sweaty heads and faces, but otherwise find it difficult to sweat. Kali phos types are usually chilly.

Common Uses
• Exhaustion • Insomnia • Jet lag
• Neuralgia • Shingles • Toothache

MODALITIES

Worse: *worry; exhaustion; overworking; cold; moving too fast; being alone*
Better: *sleeping; being warm; eating plenty; having company*

Lachesis

FULL NAME
Lachesis muta

COMMON NAME
- Surukuku snake
- Bushmaster snake

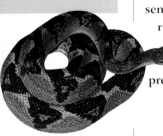

This South American reptile is a truly frightening snake, growing to 12 feet (3.5 m) long and with 1-inch (2.5 cm) fangs, a girth as thick as a man's thigh, a rainbow-coloured head and an orange body. Extremely poisonous, it is also highly aggressive, attacking at will. The bushmaster's sensitivity to vibrations and its highly developed sense of smell make it a ruthless predator. These characteristics, as well as more general snake-like traits, such as flickering tongues, form the picture of this patient. The central theme of this remedy is over-stimulation, and it is prepared from the snake's venom.

MAIN INDICATIONS

MENTAL AND EMOTIONAL

Lachesis patients are active, alert, intense, instinctive and extremely passionate. These characteristics are tainted, however, by selfishness, jealousy and venomousness.

Lachesis types generally ignore other people's needs, putting their own gratification first. However, they are very possessive of people close to them, regarding them as their property. This can lead to jealousy and suspicion. The suspicion can become obsessive until it reaches the point that they become aware of their ridiculous paranoia, making them extremely anxious. These people are constantly on the point of boiling over.

PHYSICAL

The circulation of blood forms the physical symptom picture, with high blood pressure, palpitations, flushes and varicose veins all being common. There are also septic and gangrenous complaints due to the stagnation of the blood flow.

Whenever the rhythm of circulation is affected – for example, by hormonal changes – the Lachesis picture is created. Once the blood flow normalizes, the symptoms disappear. Heat, however, generally makes the symptoms much worse because it puts huge pressure on the cardiovascular system.

Patients cannot tolerate any kind of pressure, especially from tight clothing. Headaches are bursting and the throat feels almost blocked, making swallowing very difficult; even drinks will aggravate, although hard foods can bring some relief. The symptoms start on the left.

MODALITIES

Worse: *waking; left side; spring; warm baths; pressure or constriction, especially from clothing; empty swallowing; suppressed discharges*

Better: *cold drinks; open air; discharging*

Common Uses
- Headaches • Menopause • Period pains
- Palpitations • Sore throats

Ledum

FULL NAME
Ledum palustre
(Plant family:
Ericaceae)

COMMON NAMES
• Marsh ledum
• Marsh tea
• Marsh rosemary
• Labrador tea

*L*edum palustre is most commonly found in northern countries such as Ireland, Scandinavia and Canada. The plant has a similar leaf to the rosemary bush: shiny on the upper surface with a downy underside that holds warmth. The branches are also downy towards the top but more woody near the bottom of the plant. It finds its home in boggy, marshy areas.

The plant has a long history of use because of the ledol oil it contains. The oil has antiseptic properties, making it an excellent domestic insecticide for lice and moths, as well as an effective treatment for scabies, sore throats and whooping cough.

The northern locations and physical properties of *Ledum palustre* point to the remedy's picture: patients have a feeling of coldness and a desire for solitude.

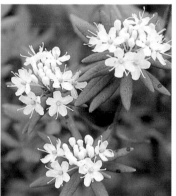

MAIN INDICATIONS

MENTAL AND EMOTIONAL

The Ledum type is angry, preferring to be left alone in order to be miserable. Ledum patients avoid people whenever possible, and in company they tend to be churlish.

PHYSICAL

Ledum is best known as a first-aid remedy for ailments such as mosquito bites and wasp stings. The affected area is extremely tender and sensitive to touch. The skin is often mottled, swollen and puffy, but feels cold – in contrast to the remedy Apis (page 24), which can also be used on such occasions. Very cold applications, such as ice, will also help relieve such afflictions, easing the stinging and itchy sensations. Heat only aggravates.

This remedy can be used to treat other injuries, such as a puncture wound from a rusty nail or crushed fingers; it has been given to help prevent tetanus. The pain is acute and feels as if it is shooting upwards. These injuries can be relieved only if the symptoms above are diagnosed, too.

Ledum is often used in cases of rheumatoid arthritis when the pain starts in the smaller joints around the fingers and toes, then moves upwards into the larger joints, with a feeling of stiffness, even burning.

Common Uses
• Wasp stings • Mosquito bites
• Puncture wounds

MODALITIES

Worse: *alcohol;
heat; movement;
night-time;
scratching*
Better: *cold
applications; rest*

Lycopodium

FULL NAME
Lycopodium clavatum
(Plant family: Lycopodiaceae)

COMMON NAMES
• Club moss
• Wolf's claw
• Lamb's tail
• Fox tail

This plant is found throughout northern Europe, especially in Russia and Finland, where it thrives on dry heaths and in pastures and woods. Its structure shares the characteristics of both moss and fern, a 'confusion' that is borne out in the emotional picture of the remedy. Lycopodium is an evergreen plant with long, trailing stems travelling far along the ground, secured by small fibred roots that look like a wolf's paw. The main bulk of the plant consists of very upright, scaly spikes, which grow in pairs and are topped by a fruit that contains tiny spores, which break down into a very light powder. It is these spores that go towards making the homoeopathic remedy.

The highly flammable nature of this powder has given rise to Lycopodium being referred to as 'vegetable sulphur', and it was used in Germany to manufacture fireworks and by theatres to produce the effect of lightning. The powder is incredibly fine, tasteless and odourless, with an amazing resistance to water. It is said that if you put your hand in a glass of water that has the powder sprinkled on top, you can reach the bottom of the glass without getting your hand wet.

MAIN INDICATIONS

MENTAL AND EMOTIONAL

To understand Lycopodium types we must first understand the extreme lack of confidence that lurks within them, producing a very deep sense of cowardliness. Most of the symptoms that we see on the emotional level are about the ways in which they overcompensate for what they perceive as a great weakness.

The feelings of inadequacy make Lycopodium types feel incapable of fulfilling any responsibilities, so they try to avoid such situations if they possibly can. They are skilled at bluffing their way through things and often take on an air of extreme haughtiness, arrogance and pretension to hide their inadequacies. They can be intellectually very astute, although physically they are fairly inactive.

Lycopodium patients hate weakness in others simply because it reminds them of their own failings. They may even bully others who are weaker than them. This inflates their own ego, giving them a much-needed sense of strength and power. The thing the Lycopodium patient dreads most is being exposed for what they are: weak.

Relationships and responsibility are two very difficult words in the

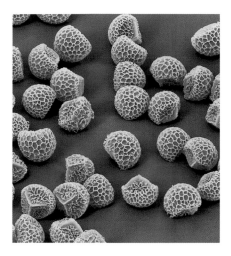

Lycopodium vocabulary, especially in terms of commitment. There is a strong desire for sexual gratification, but such people are more comfortable with one-night stands. Once they are in a relationship, huge problems can occur regarding sexual dysfunction and impotence, leading to further feelings of inadequacy. They would generally rather flee from the relationship than work through the problems, or they will be horribly dictatorial and tyrannical within the home (where the threat is) and delightful outside it.

PHYSICAL

The inflated ego is also expressed here through windy digestive symptoms, and 95% of Lycopodium cases are thought to have gastro-intestinal problems, exposing weaknesses. Both flatulence and bloating occur, especially after eating. Patients can feel incredibly full after eating a tiny amount of food and yet are often the sort to over-indulge,

in keeping with their constant need for gratification. They love sweet things and oysters, both of which are terribly bad for them. In this way Lycopodium types can be contrasted with Nux vomica types (page 80) who over-indulge for reasons of stress and tension within the digestive system. Liver problems are often indicated in the Lycopodium picture, which has great relevance as emotionally the liver is associated with cowardice. Jaundice and constipation follow as a result.

Many of these patients' complaints are on the right side or will begin on the right side and then move to the left. There is also a strongly defined time of aggravation between 4 and 8 p.m. when they are much worse, as well as invariably feeling dreadful on waking due to a sluggish liver.

There is an unusual symptom that one foot may feel cold and the other hot. Warm, stuffy rooms only aggravate matters, leading patients to stick their feet out of the bed to get some air or simply to cool them down.

Lycopodium patients' appearance can be quite telling. They frequently have quite a sallow complexion with flushed cheeks and a red nose. The forehead is often wrinkled, and they may appear old before their time, going prematurely grey, perhaps. The body can look lean, even emaciated, with poor muscle tone.

Common Uses

• Flatulence • Indigestion • Anxiety

MODALITIES

Worse: *tight clothing (especially around the waist); heat; waking up; flatulence; oysters; over-indulgence; indigestion; late afternoon, evening; lying on the right side*

Better: *warm drinks; warm food; cold applications; motion; burping; urinating; loosening the clothes; cool or open air*

FULL NAME
Magnesia phosphorica

SOURCE
• Phosphate of magnesium

Mag phos

Mag phos is one of twelve homoeopathic remedies present in the tissues of the body and known collectively as tissue salts. It can also be found in cereals, oranges, grapefruit, beer and lettuce. The remedy is made by combining magnesium sulphate with sodium phosphate to form crystals.

MAIN INDICATIONS

MENTAL AND EMOTIONAL

Mag phos types feel so much pain that they often find it difficult to think straight, and they may talk obsessively about the pain to the exclusion of any other subject. They feel exhausted and can become tearful very easily. Generally, they love to communicate with people but are often cautious of what they say in case they say the wrong thing and are no longer liked. This can become so extreme that they may withdraw altogether and have a fear of people. Mag phos types tend to be thin, nervous and highly strung.

PHYSICAL

Mag phos is one of the great remedies for treating spasmodic pain throughout the body. We see an array of different pains, although characteristically they are sharp, shooting, cramping pains, and they are almost always soothed by heat and massage.

It can be an heroic remedy for painful periods. Those who experience agonizing pain on a monthly basis and who find that the only cure is to curl up with a hot-water bottle and gently massage the abdomen may find great relief from this remedy. The pain in a Mag phos situation can be so extreme as to cause the patient to vomit.

Digestive cramps are also helped by the use of this remedy. Likewise, flatulent colic with intense griping pains, which cause the patient to bend double but are better for warmth and massage, can also be helped by the use of Mag phos. The abdomen can feel extremely bloated, but passing wind does not relieve the pain. There may be a desire to walk around while passing wind, and all the clothes need to be loosened in a quest for comfort. When moving around, dizziness may be experienced, as well as a tendency to fall forwards.

Cramps associated with prolonged or continual use of parts of the body are also a common feature of the Mag phos picture. In writer's cramp, for example, the fingers can just suddenly give out and become too painful to use. Again the pains will be sharp, cramping and shooting, but relieved by warmth and gentle massage.

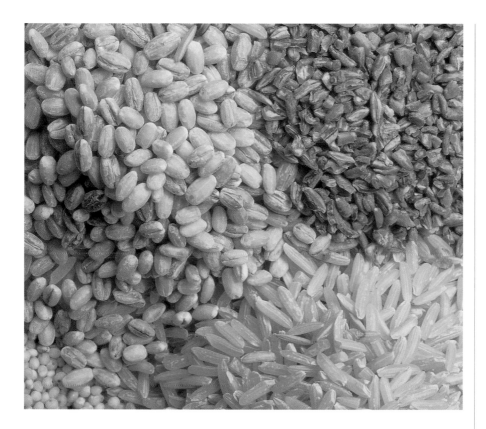

It is a great remedy for neuralgia where the pain shoots along the nerves or along the spine. The nerves can feel as if they have been torn. Any form of coldness will aggravate the condition.

Headaches helped by Mag phos are those that throb and pulsate, not dissimilar to those in the Belladonna picture (page 34). Tight headwear, such as bandages or a hat, can be used to create pressure around the head, which may ease the pain.

Mag phos is a good remedy for neuralgic toothaches, when the pain shoots along the nerve and is aggravated by cold drinks and cold air but relieved by anything warm. Similarly, it is an effective treatment for painful teething in babies and infants.

In acute asthma attacks Mag phos may help relax the spasms in the chest, calming the situation. The cough of Mag phos tends to be dry and tickling and worsened by lying down but eased by cool air. This remedy is also useful in easing the spasmodic coughing of whooping cough.

Common Uses

- Period pains • Colic • Neuralgia
- Post-labour pains • Toothache

MODALITIES

Worse: *cold things; being cold*
Better: *warmth; gentle massage; bending forwards*

FULL NAME
Mercurius solubilis

COMMON NAME
• Quicksilver

Merc sol

Mercurius solubilis is the ammonium nitrate salt of mercury. It is an intensely poisonous substance, with the symptoms having a close similarity to the disease syphilis. Mercury has been used medicinally since the fifteenth century and was used extensively in the treatment of venereal disease.

Mercury, commonly known as quicksilver, easily scatters into tiny globules and is extremely destructive in its nature. Looking at mercury in its raw state and seeing the damage that it can do make's it possible to gain an understanding of this remedy's homoeopathic uses.

MAIN INDICATIONS

MENTAL AND EMOTIONAL

Thinking of the scattered nature of mercury we can understand the instability that is so strongly indicated in these types. They are intensely changeable and sensitive; like the mercury in a thermometer that reacts to every slight change in temperature, mercury patients react acutely on an emotional level to their environment.

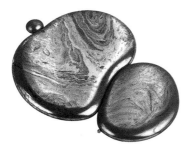

The outside world seems full of hostility to Merc sol patients, and paranoia about other people is extreme, punctuated by the thought that nearly everyone is an enemy. Merc sol types are usually suspicious and cautious, and they may frequently appear hurried and restless.

The mind may become increasingly confused, leading to a gradual but destructive breakdown. Their sense of self-identity is lacking and they can be fearful of becoming mad – one of the final stages of syphilis.

Little of what they fear is expressed, except in sudden outbursts, which are often very violent in nature, even to the extent of wanting to kill. They feel lonely and isolated, and self-disgust is prominent. They need to try to create stability in an increasingly unstable world. The contradiction of their own emotions causes increasing debility.

PHYSICAL

As on the emotional level, destruction is very apparent here, and we see a lack of stability, especially where temperature is concerned. Patients are increasingly sensitive to any temperature change, which can immediately lead to physical dysfunction.

Offensiveness is also a keynote within this remedy, with a great many foul discharges, such as perspiration, pus and stools, which all flow freely. Sweating is especially prominent; usually occurring all over the body; it can often smell rancid and even stain the sheets.

Merc sol patients frequently suffer with ulceration, and in mercury we find one of the best remedies for mouth ulcers. There are copious amounts of saliva, accompanied by a strange metallic taste, the tongue appears flabby and flaccid, possibly showing teeth imprints. Gums may bleed easily, and the teeth are often in poor condition, sometimes discoloured, black and loose. Abscesses on the gums are also common and are usually accompanied by excessive saliva and foul-smelling breath.

The throat can be extremely sore, with the pain extending up to the ears. There may be a constant desire to swallow, in spite of the pain. The tonsils are often inflamed, ulcerated, suppurating and bluish-red in colour. The glands can become swollen, with stitching pains that extend to the ear when swallowing.

The patient can have extensive amounts of infected catarrh in the case of sinusitis, which also makes the mouth taste horrible. The catarrh is usually green or yellow in colour and smells offensive, like old cheese. The infected discharges may burn the upper lip and make the nostrils raw and ulcerated.

Mercury is a good remedy for diarrhoea. The stools are often extremely offensive to smell, burning and watery, and sometimes green or yellow in colour. They may become slimy and blood stained in extreme cases. Mercury patients often have a feeling of great exhaustion after passing stools and a feeling as if they haven't quite finished, with a burning sensation continuing after the stool has left the body.

Most Merc sol patients are often extremely thirsty, despite the copious amounts of saliva that they produce. They also have a strange food desire for bread and butter. In addition, Merc sol is one of the main remedies for ulcerative colitis.

All the symptoms of this remedy are much worse at night.

Common Uses

• Mouth ulcers • Diarrhoea • Fever
• Sore throat • Sinusitis

MODALITIES

Worse: *night-time; sweating; lying on the right side; over-heating; temperature change; getting the feet wet*

Better: *moderate temperature; resting; in the morning*

Nat mur

Salt is found in great abundance in our bodies and the food we eat. It consists of two quite harmful elements, sodium and chlorine, which are relatively safe once combined, however. Salt aids our fluid balance but can also make us ill if we have too much or too little – for example, in Addison's disease symptoms of overwhelming irritability and lethargy occur due to poor salt balance. If someone's salt intake is too high numerous problems will occur, including inflammation, urticaria (rashes), wart formations, dry skin and loss of hair.

These are all symptoms we see in Nat mur patients. The ease with which our salt balance can fluctuate gives us huge polarities in this picture, which is indicated by the different natures of sodium and chloride. It is these differing polarities, or 'natures', that are found in the Nat mur patient.

Another close association with salt is, of course, the sea, which covers 60% of the earth's surface and is thus a major part of our environment. Our relationship with water and the sea is often emotional, which is strongly reflected in the emotional picture of Nat mur.

MAIN INDICATIONS

MENTAL AND EMOTIONAL

Nat mur is often referred to as a 'very British remedy'. The picture is aptly described by the words of the song 'I am a Rock' by Simon and Garfunkel, which includes the phrases 'I am an island', 'I am alone', 'I build walls' and 'No one touches me', which all reflect the Nat mur picture. It is this initial sensitivity and vulnerability that plays such an important role.

Grief, hurt or humiliation can inflict intense pain, causing a shut-down of patients' emotional centres, as it seems to strike right at the heart. They will build walls around themselves and aim to control any emotions. As a result, you will find individuals who seem very cold and closed, who rarely cry and who cannot bear to be consoled. Despite all this, however, there is a huge desire for love and emotional attachment. They care greatly for the welfare of others, often choosing a caring profession.

Nat mur patients like to wallow in self-pity, which is often accompanied by thoughts of the past and makes them retreat into their own world. The ability to love may show itself through fantasy, when feelings are not real or feasible, thus exacerbating any feelings of rejection and hurt. The one thing that may change this state of affairs is alcohol: a surprisingly chatty and rather lewd character may appear after a bottle of wine. This appals the Nat mur type, who will quickly harden as the sun comes up.

There is a hysterical side to this remedy, which is rarely seen but may come as a final resort if the suppression is too extreme. It is revealed in response to harsh criticism or a reprimand.

PHYSICAL

Many physical symptoms will appear after a long period of introversion, which may have been brought on by death or a failed relationship. Patients can have extreme sensitivity to noise, touch and, in particular, light. Nat mur patients find sunlight quite difficult, especially the heat of the sun, which often brings on intense, periodical migraines or headaches that are bursting and hammering and intolerant of any movement. The worst time of day for these types is between 10 a.m. and 3 p.m.

Nat mur patients are prone to frequent colds, with profuse discharges of clear, watery mucus that resembles egg white. The mucus may drip down the back of the throat, tasting bitter and salty. This may alternate with a stuffed-up feeling in the nose that makes breathing very difficult and may affect the ability to taste and smell. There is often a watery discharge from the eyes, and profuse sneezing is common.

Depression and mood swings can lead to a state of hypochondria; a patient may become obsessive about cleaning and disinfecting in an attempt to ward off germs. They may be especially scared of heart disease – their most hidden and sacred chamber.

There is a water imbalance within this remedy, and patients will often have an immense thirst. However, there is a huge craving for salt, which inevitably leads to this sense of dryness. Cold sores and warts are common, and the skin will often become dry and cracked. Patients are also prone to getting blisters on the tip of the tongue. Furthering the association with salt and water, Nat mur patients either love or hate the sea.

Nat mur patients tend to be chilly, and yet they dislike heat and being in a stuffy atmosphere.

Common Uses

- Depression • Grief • Headaches
- Cold sores

MODALITIES

Worse: *in the morning; heat; sun; sympathy; puberty; crying; recurring malaria; lying down; overwhelming emotion*

Better: *open air; cool bathing; sweating; seashore; fasting*

Nat sulph

FULL NAME
Natrum
sulphuricum

SOURCE
• Glauberite

Nat sulph is made from sodium sulphate, which is isolated from the mineral glauberite. Found in many spa waters, it is one of twelve homoeopathic remedies that are present in the tissues of the body and are known as tissue salts.

MAIN INDICATIONS

MENTAL AND EMOTIONAL

As with all Natrum remedy pictures, we see elements of being closed and shut down. Nat sulph types are individuals who feel a tremendous sense of responsibility. They are down to earth, hard working and realistic about life. They almost sacrifice their own needs for the sense of duty that they feel, which can close them off from their real emotional state. They can feel neglected, are rarely expressive and are estranged from their own family, almost as if their heart has been locked away. Deep depression, lack of joy and suicidal feelings may also be experienced, while soft music and lighting may move them to tears.

PHYSICAL

Nat sulph is a great remedy after head injuries. Patients may experience a change in their mental or physical condition, with memory loss and irritability, or tinnitus and vertigo.

Symptoms are aggravated by cold and damp: either wet weather or places. As autumn approaches their hearts sink. It is a particularly useful remedy for asthma, if attacks are triggered by dampness.

The cough is rattling and sits deep in the chest, often producing thick, ropy and greenish-yellow sputum. The lungs feel uncomfortably devoid of air, forcing the patient to sit up and hold their chest. Diarrhoea, bloatedness and nausea may all be present, together with a bitter taste in the mouth and a green-coated tongue.

The liver region may feel particularly sensitive, usually in the morning, once the patient has got out of bed. Nat sulph is known as a liverish remedy, helping to eliminate toxicity from the body. It is good for hangovers and can be a helpful remedy as part of a 'spring-clean' programme.

MODALITIES

Worse: *damp, wet weather and surroundings; head injuries; autumn and spring; fatty foods*
Better: *dry weather and surroundings; sitting up*

Common Uses
• Nausea • Asthma • Diarrhoea
• Hangovers

Nit ac

FULL NAME
Nitricum acidum

SOURCE
• Nitric acid

Nitric acid is a colourless, corrosive acid that is commonly used in the manufacture of such disparate things as fertilizers and explosives. It has been used medicinally as a tonic for hundreds of years, which is why it is also sometimes known as aqua fortis.

MAIN INDICATIONS

MENTAL AND EMOTIONAL

Nit ac types feel very discontented with their lot, highly dissatisfied and cross with themselves. They are angry and irritable, and this can extend to others, especially to those who have let them down or offended them in some way. When this happens, they are reluctant to accept any apologies offered, meeting them instead with obstinacy and stubbornness. They can feel vindictive and vengeful, while pitying themselves immensely.

The basis for these symptoms can be explained by a wearing down of the emotions from long-term caring or nursing of others, where the patient's own needs have been set aside. An emotional reaction to physical exhaustion from lack of sleep may also be a cause. They can be extremely anxious about their own health and have a particular fear of cancer.

PHYSICAL

Weakness is prevalent in this picture: these patients have burned themselves out. All discharges are watery, acrid, foul and bloody, with a sour and unpleasant smell. Ulceration can develop in the mouth, throat, eyes, genitalia and anus. These situations are characterized by splintering and stitch-like pains. Sore throats are another feature, together with the ulceration in the mouth, and the breath can smell quite unpleasant.

This remedy also helps fissures of the anus when the rectum feels torn, as with haemorrhoids, which may be itchy or burning or bleed easily. There is also a violent cutting, lingering pain during and after the stool.

The corrosive action of Nit ac makes it an excellent remedy for warts, which are often jagged and bleed easily. Patients feel chilly, but feel much better when travelling in a car. Symptoms are aggravated at night, especially just after midnight. They also have a particular love of fatty and salty foods.

Common Uses
• Sore throats • Ulcers • Haemorrhoids
• Warts

MODALITIES

Worse: *night-time;*
cold; lack of sleep;
jarring
Better: *being warm;*
travelling in a car

Nux vomica

FULL NAME
*Strychnos
nux-vomica*
(Plant family:
Loganiaceae)

COMMON NAME
• Poison nut

*S***trychnos nux-vomica** is a tree found mainly in the East Indies, the Malay archipelago and northern Australia. Small, with a crooked trunk and knotted new growth, the tree has smooth, ash-coloured bark and large, oval-shaped, shiny leaves. The flowers, which blossom in the cold season, are small, green-white and funnel-shaped, with a very unpleasant odour. The fruit is a beautiful orange-coloured globe, about the size of an apple, with a hard rind. Inside is a soft, pulpy, white jelly, which holds five seeds from which we obtain the remedy: they contain a lethal cocktail, including alkaloids and strychnine.

Alkaloid strychnine poisoning has a profound effect on the whole nervous system. Poisoning begins with difficulty in breathing, acute anxiety and twitching, followed by horrific seizures. The seizures can be so violent that the head is forced back as far as the buttocks, causing the spine to break. The spasms may cease for a while, but the sensitivity of the nervous system becomes so extreme that the slightest noise can bring on further, more intense spasms. Death usually occurs from exhaustion.

MAIN INDICATIONS

MENTAL AND EMOTIONAL

Nux vomica types live on their nerves, are irritable and can display anger that is impulsive, usually resulting from a strong reaction to their environment. They are acutely sensitive to all external impressions – smell, noise, draughts and so on – and this is sometimes referred to as the picture of city-dwellers, where life always seems non-stop. Nux vomica types are, typically, workaholics who live off adrenaline and stimulants. They may be the 'road rage' maniacs, who become violent and angry at others on the road. They are highly ambitious and need to be the best – nothing else will do. Their desire to achieve is so enormous that they become extremely frustrated at anything that gets in their way and so are very fastidious and fault-finding. Imagine a hangover – this is an example of the Nux vomica state: quarrelsome, looking for a fight and enraged by the slightest noise. Nux vomica types can be so angry that they have an impulse to kill. They can also have a strong sense of social injustice, coupled with a great need to be independent. They find intimacy quite difficult, leading to difficulties when accepting comfort from another – they refuse to be consoled.

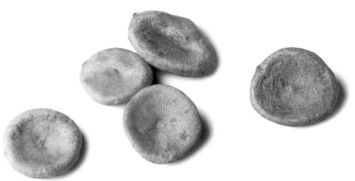

Anxiety, stemming from stress, can be quite acute, and there is a need for order, tidiness and accuracy. These feelings and emotions are very exhausting, hence the need for vast quantities of coffee and, perhaps, several drinks after work – none of which help their physical state.

PHYSICAL

In the Nux vomica picture, spasms and tensions within the body are rife. Just as we see in strychnine poisonings, there will be a profusely cramped state. This is especially true of gastric complaints, when indigestion causes cramping and the waist feels constricted by clothes that must be loosened immediately. Pain in the stomach usually occurs 2–3 hours after eating and may be accompanied by nausea and wind.

Constipation is common in Nux vomica types, and there is a great urge to defecate and yet nothing happens, but when they relax the stool comes. However, there is often a feeling as if they haven't quite finished. The peristaltic action is sometimes reversed, and they may go to pass a stool only to suddenly find that they are nauseous instead.

Sleep patterns can suffer badly, and they often wake in the early morning – between 3 and 4 a.m., the 'liver time'. At this time the symptoms do not seem to be that bad, but once the patient wakes up later on in the morning, they are much worse.

Headaches often feel like 'hangover headaches', when the pain is either at the back of the head or lying heavily over one eye. There is an extreme sensitivity to light or noise, with a loathing of food and tobacco smoke. The patient feels fuzzy and confused, and the only relief comes from the pressure of a warm hand.

There will be a huge craving for stimulants, and comfort foods. Nux vomica patients tend to be very chilly, disliking open air and cold in general; all their pains are better for heat.

Common Uses

- Constipation • Nausea • Indigestion
- Flatulence • Headaches • Hangovers
- Insomnia

MODALITIES

Worse: *early in the morning; being cold; over-indulgence; sedentary habits; mental exertion; disturbed sleep; pressure of clothes; noise; light; touch; smell*

Better: *taking naps; pressure on the head; hot drinks; warm rooms; evenings; after defecating; loosening of clothes*

Opium

FULL NAME
Papaver somniferum
(Plant family:
Papaveraceae)

COMMON NAME
• Opium poppy

Opium is a highly addictive drug, and it has been used through the centuries, both for recreational purposes and, in the medical world, as a painkiller and sleep-inducer. The seeds produce a milky fluid, which is dried and rolled into balls. Opium contains many alkaloids, and it is from this plant that morphine and heroin are obtained.

MAIN INDICATIONS

MENTAL AND EMOTIONAL

In the Opium picture we find types with a disturbed state of consciousness. Their sense of reality and their ability to assess their environment are diminished, leaving them unable to make sound judgements. They have an indifference to both pleasure and pain, and they may often feel withdrawn from life, saying that they are fine when, to the observer, they are obviously not. They can also appear overly excited, even overcome by a delirious state, with strange delusions and wide, staring eyes. They can act in a dangerous or thoughtless way as they have no sense of the consequences.

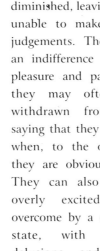

Many of the symptoms in this remedy will stem from some form of shock, such as a sudden fright, bereavement or disappointment.

PHYSICAL

On a physical level, Opium types show a strange painlessness, when one would normally expect pain. There is a lack of reaction and activity on all levels, and patients seem weak, slow, dull and drowsy, as if in a stupor. They have lost their power and self-control.

This remedy is useful after head injuries when sleepiness continues for a long period of time: patients may feel sleepy but are unable to sleep, due to an acute sensitivity to noise. When they finally do sleep, respiration is disturbed. Their breathing can sound heavy and laboured, commonly coupled with heavy snoring. They feel incredibly hot and will sweat profusely. Constipation is common, and there may be urine retention as well, although stools or urine may be passed involuntarily if they experience shock.

Common Uses
• Concussion • Constipation • Shock
• Injury • Sleep problems

MODALITIES

Worse: *shock;
fright; heat;
during sleep*
Better: *being in the
open air; cold*

Phos ac

FULL NAME
Phosphoric acid

This substance is made from ground bones and sulphuric acid. Its acid nature gives it a strong affinity with the nervous system.

MAIN INDICATIONS

MENTAL AND EMOTIONAL

Phos ac is an excellent remedy for the exhaustion and debility that stem from any emotional cause. The main characteristic of Phos ac types is their overwhelming need for contact. If this precious contact is broken, moreover, a breakdown in the ability to communicate will follow shortly. Depression, exhaustion and, perhaps, indifference are often triggered when someone emotionally close to them dies or moves away.

Phos ac is a good remedy for homesickness, grief and disappointed love – feelings that are all expressed by shutting down and closing off from the outside world. There may be a strong level of indifference when nothing matters anymore, nothing is of any interest and the patient becomes introspective and has no desire to talk. Familiar things may seem alien to them, well-known details escape their mind, and they answer slowly and often incorrectly when asked questions. They feel unclear, hazy and pessimistic about life.

Indifference can also be seen after long periods of studying or taxing mental work, when their brainpower and nervous system feel drained and the ability to think no longer exists.

PHYSICAL

The weakness that is felt on an emotional level is also expressed in the physical body. The immune system is low, and patients can catch colds very easily. It is a good remedy to aid recovery after a long period of illness, when weakness sets in due to loss of fluids, from sweating or urinating, for example. Surprisingly, patients can feel better after a bout of diarrhoea, which often indicates the beginning of the recovery process. Because of the weakness experienced, sexual indifference may occur, together with impotence and debility as a result of the loss of seminal fluids. Hair loss and early greying after grief are also common.

Phos ac types often feel dehydrated and have a desire for juicy, fresh things, and fizzy drinks, while remaining averse to sour foods.

Common Uses
• Exhaustion • Debility • Grief

MODALITIES

Worse: *cold;*
loss of fluids;
over-studying;
emotional grief
and loss
Better: *diarrhoea;*
catnaps; warmth

FULL NAME
Phosphorus, the element

COMMON NAME
• White phosphorus

Phosphorus

Phosphorus is an essential element in life, helping with the transfer of energy within plant cells through chemical reactions. It is highly combustible at room temperature and must be stored in water or alcohol.

Unlike sulphur, which homoeopaths believe acts in accordance with the force of gravity, phosphorus rises up into the atmosphere and seems to disappear completely. This easy diffusion is important when looking at the remedy Phosphorus.

The poisoning picture of the Phosphorus state is extraordinary. There are many burning pains, with vomit often containing luminous blood. The liver is particularly affected, as are the tissues of the mucous membranes, where inflammation is widespread, eventually leading to haemorrhaging and, possibly, anaemia. The nervous system becomes hypersensitive and excitable.

MAIN INDICATIONS

MENTAL AND EMOTIONAL

Like the element itself, Phosphorus is all about diffusion. There is a very easy flow of energy, emotion and awareness, with few or no barriers. Phosphorus characters are open to all influences, and they exude an enormous amount of warmth, expression, affection and sensitivity. They have a considerable amount of artistic and musical talent, which is expressed with intelligence and delicacy.

Both strangers and friends are extremely important and will receive a great deal of affection from the Phosphorus type. Unlike the remedies Sulphur (page 98) and Arsenicum (page 30), communication takes the form of a genuine care for others, with the ego playing only a small part. Their vulnerability to external influences means that Phosphorus patients can be impressionable but at the same time easily reassured. There is a great deal of activity in their heads and they feel easily 'spaced out', as if floating. The resulting effect is of being easily startled, when a sudden noise, such as a clap of thunder, brings them back down to earth with a bump.

Phosphorus patients also tend to be fearful because of their sensitivity. They can fear the dark or being alone. Their concern for others gives them immense anticipatory fears, with genuine anxiety for friends. In more advanced stages the fears can be quite overwhelming, occupying their minds more and more, to the extent that their respiratory system may suffer, causing hyperventilation. They begin to fear death, especially from cancer, and they may start to have a sensation of bubbles in their body, as if they are lightweight and could easily float away.

Sleep comes easily for Phosphorus patients; they find it easy to drift off, and even a quick nap will often leave them refreshed. In the latter stages of the remedy, however, sleep may become difficult, and they will wake feeling tense and nervy. In extreme cases, the mind can break down completely, and a feeling of utter indifference may result.

PHYSICAL

Phosphorus types can bleed easily – even the blood has no barriers – and nosebleeds, bleeding gums and ulcers will all be common. The menses will be profuse and prolonged.

All symptoms will appear quickly; colds will start in the head and rapidly move down the throat to the chest. There is great hoarseness of the voice, together with a constant desire to clear the throat. The chest feels tight, and any coughing will be hard, dry and exhausting, arising from a change in temperature. There may also be a sense of burning in the lungs. Sputum may be blood streaked and rusty in colour, and lying down, especially on the left side, will make the coughing worse.

Phosphorus types often have a ravenous hunger and may suffer from

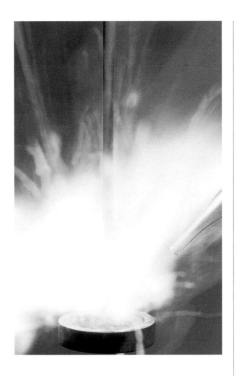

hypoglycaemia. Burning pains in the stomach are accompanied by an enormous thirst for cold water. This brings great relief until the water becomes warm in the stomach, when the need to vomit will return again.

Phosphorus is a particularly useful remedy for nausea and exhaustion after an anaesthetic. Energy levels can burn out very easily, and exhaustion is rife. But even when they are unwell, the Phosphorus patient can have bright, sparkling eyes and a fresh, ruddy complexion.

Common Uses

- Bronchitis • Gastroenteritis • Nosebleeds
- Operations • Vomiting

MODALITIES

Worse: *lying on the left side; cold; warm food and drinks; mental fatigue; changing weather*

Better: *eating; sleeping; cold food and water; sitting up; lying on the right side*

Phytolacca

FULL NAME
Phytolacca americana
(Plant family: Phytolaccaceae)

COMMON NAME
• Poke root

Phytolacca is found growing in damp ground in eastern North America. It has a smooth, purple-green stem that grows to about 3 feet (1 m) high and pointed, oval leaves and green-white flowers. The dark purple berries are highly poisonous and cause agonizing, griping pains in the stomach, followed by severe vomiting, which can lead to physical jerking, a sore throat, a congested face and swollen tonsils. Historically, the plant was used for cattle with lumpy udders that produced little milk. All these symptoms give a strong idea of what to expect from this remedy.

MAIN INDICATIONS

MENTAL AND EMOTIONAL
Phytolacca types show an indifference to life, despite being terrified that they might die, and any pain can feel unbearable.

PHYSICAL
Phytolacca, which is known as 'the vegetable mercury', has many similarities to Merc Sol (page 74): there is a soreness that pervades the whole body, with shooting pains that suddenly appear and disappear. Phytolacca is a helpful remedy for any breast-related ailments, when the breasts feel stony-hard and swollen, and very tender. They are particularly painful during breast-feeding, and the pain can send spasms all over the body. Hard nodules may be present in the breasts, which have a tendency to suppurate and ulcerate. The nipples are often cracked and sore and can continue to produce a bloody, watery discharge long after breast-feeding has finished.

The throat symptoms are numerous. This is a remedy for recurrent or acute tonsillitis where the tonsils look dark red (in contrast to the bright red of Belladonna (page 34)) with white spots. The pain is usually aggravated by such things as warm drinks, but in general, the patient is worse for being in cold or damp situations. The throat may feel dry, rough and full, making swallowing very painful, but the urge to swallow remains strong. The glands are swollen, and pain extends from the throat to the ear. Any mucus present is tough and stringy and difficult to remove.

All these symptoms can be helped by clenching the teeth.

Common Uses
• Breast-feeding • Mastitis • Tonsillitis
• Sore throat

MODALITIES
Worse: *motion; night-time; cold; damp; breast-feeding; hot drinks; swallowing*
Better: *cold drinks; rest; warmth; dry weather; holding breasts*

Podophyllum

Podophyllum is a herb found growing in North America in damp, wet meadows. It has a single, sickly-smelling white flower, which blooms in May but then drops off, only to be succeeded by a red fruit. North American Indians found Podophyllum very useful for purging poisons from the body.

FULL NAME
Podophyllum
peltatum
(Plant family:
Berberidaceae)

COMMON NAMES
• American mandrake
• May apple
• May flower

MAIN INDICATIONS

MENTAL AND EMOTIONAL

Sadness and depression dominate this remedy: it is mainly used in acute situations when patients feel that they may die or that everything in their life seems wrong. They are extremely tired, but they feel restless and fidgety.

PHYSICAL

It is the digestive system that is so highly disturbed in this remedy. The stomach gurgles and rumbles, and intense cramping pains can cause the patient to double up in agony. The abdomen feels sore and tender, and any pressure or touch will exacerbate the problem.

Once the pain has set in, spluttering and foul-smelling diarrhoea follows. The cramping pains usually disappear after the diarrhoea, but may soon return, in time for the next bout.

There is an 'all gone' sensation in the stomach, as if both it and the abdomen are being dragged downwards. Patients often lose their appetite, despite a gnawing hunger. A headache, which is related to the digestive disturbance, may accompany the illness. The head feels as if it will burst open, especially at the back, but is relieved once the diarrhoea has passed. Patients may want to vomit profusely, and this will, unfortunately, end in an ejection of yellow bile.

Any diarrhoea that occurs during menstruation will be accompanied by a sore uterus and a dragging down feeling of the organs. Patients will feel totally exhausted and may also excrete offensive sweat. Summer heat can be a cause, as can teething in a child, and all symptoms will generally be worse in the early morning.

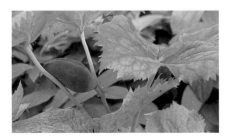

Common Uses
• Diarrhoea • Gastroenteritis

MODALITIES

Worse: *bathing;*
summertime;
early morning;
teething
Better: *lying on the*
stomach; bending
forwards; warmth

Pulsatilla

FULL NAME
Pulsatilla pratensis
(Plant family:
Ranunculaceae)

COMMON NAMES
• Windflower
• Meadow
  anemone
• Pasque flower

Pulsatilla is a small, beautiful European plant that grows most happily in a chalk soil. The plant grows to about 8 inches (20 cm) in height, with fern-like leaves and has bell-shaped, rich purple flowers that have a golden centre. The lovely flowers are borne on silky-soft stems, and below each flower is a ruff of hairy leaves. These plants are unobtrusive and tend to grow quietly in the company of each other.

The smell of the crushed flowers can cause bad headaches, fainting fits and inflammation to the eyes. Pulsatilla flowers have been used extensively for centuries: it is said that wise men and magicians used to pick the flowers in early spring and wrap them in red cloth to wear around their necks in case their medicinal powers were needed urgently. The whole plant is used to make the homoeopathic remedy.

MAIN INDICATIONS

MENTAL AND EMOTIONAL

Patients using this remedy have a great need for company. Pulsatilla children will be insecure without their parents around or, if the parents are present, the children will cling desperately to them for fear of being deserted. This fear of abandonment can also bring out emotions of jealousy and aggression, something that is shown particularly clearly when a new sibling is born or, with adults, if an old lover finds someone new. Tears can occur frequently and at the drop of a hat, but are easily stopped with expressions of love and solid reassurance.

There is a great need for approval within Pulsatilla types, and they will adapt themselves to give what they feel is needed for the love and affection they desire. However, this makes them easy targets for abuse and manipulation by those they need most.

Shyness and timidity are acute, especially with strangers, and patients will develop a dislike for large crowds, feeling that their security and safety are threatened. Their timidity makes them blush easily, and they are often softly spoken, preferring not to show anger and aggression.

Changeability is another key word within this picture: patients can prove to be quite moody, sulky and pouty, and yet they are very intolerant of change in others, as this again compromises their feeling of security. It is a remedy that is often called for during puberty, the stage of personal development with the greatest changes, and conversely the one that reflects the most reluctance for change, especially from the comfort and security of childhood. The patient may revert to bed-wetting and thumb-sucking in times of trauma.

The heart rather than the head rules Pulsatilla types. Emotionally, they are expressive and enjoy deep intimacy with others. They communicate tearfully, especially when telling others their symptoms, but crying makes them feel much better.

There is also a fanatical and dogmatic tendency within the Pulsatilla psyche. Because of their inability to think clearly and believe in themselves, patients may adhere strongly to ideas imposed upon them by others. This fanatical side is usually seen at a deeper stage of pathology.

PHYSICAL

Pulsatilla types feel the cold, yet have an extreme intolerance to heat. They must have fresh air and prefer to sleep with the windows open.

Their symptoms may change frequently, reflecting the changeability on the emotional level of this remedy. Pain will wander about the body as if it cannot decide where to be.

Copious discharge will flow from the eyes, nose and ears, differing in type and colour. Nasal catarrh can be also be chronic, together with profuse discharges during the day and a blocked sensation at night-time. These feelings will be relieved once the

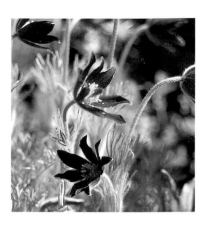

patient is removed from warm, stuffy surroundings.

The digestive system is one of the main areas of disturbance. This is not helped by a desire for rich, fatty foods, which will have a bad effect on the patient. Stomach pains usually occur a few hours after eating, with a sensation of bloatedness and heaviness. A dry mouth and headaches will also present problems, in conjunction with the digestive symptoms.

As with Nux vomica (page 80), there can be both constipation and violent, burning diarrhoea. Any vomiting is often caused by an emotional upset or from getting too excited.

Ear problems are also prominent, especially in children. Otitis media is common and there can be hearing impairment from catarrh in the eustachian tubes.

The patient may experience complications with menstruation, and general feelings of being unwell since puberty. Pulsatilla is also an excellent remedy during pregnancy, particularly if the baby is in the breech position.

Pulsatilla patients can appear delicate, fair and sweet looking, with a tendency to being plump.

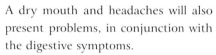

Common Uses
- Conjunctivitis • Earache • Catarrh
- Diarrhoea • Gastritis • Headaches

MODALITIES

Worse: *being too warm; wet feet; in the evening; beginning of motion; lying on left side; eating rich foods; pregnancy; puberty; during menses*

Better: *cold; fresh open air; gentle motion; crying; cold drinks and food; hard pressure*

FULL NAME
Rhus toxicodendron
(Plant family:
Anacardiaceae)

COMMON NAME
• Poison ivy

Rhus tox

Poison ivy is mainly found on the east coast of North America, particularly in Canada, as a shrub or a woody vine, which meanders restlessly, constantly spreading itself. The roots trail along the ground and are the most poisonous part of the plant. The leaves are enticingly glossy green, with hints of crimson, and the fruit grows in clusters of small, smooth, ivory-coloured berries. The remedy is made from freshly gathered leaves, picked after sunset, or on a cloudy day, from shady places.

Poison ivy dermatitis is an unpleasant allergic reaction, consisting of small, intensely itchy spots, which spread to the mucous membranes: the throat and mouth may swell, causing nausea, vomiting and an irritating cough; the joints will become painful and stiff.

MAIN INDICATIONS

MENTAL AND EMOTIONAL
Rhus tox is a despondent type, full of cares and worries. Patients are tormented by unpleasant thoughts, constantly concerned for the future, their family and business. Their thinking can be rigid, and they can seem cold and unemotional, incapable of spontaneous warmth and expression. They will feel restless internally, irritated by their physical stiffness, and highly impatient.

PHYSICAL
Themes of rigidity and restlessness are continued here, with rheumatic pain causing swollen, stiff, aching joints, which can even feel bruised and numb. The pain is the same after an injury, such as a sprained ankle, and it gets worse in damp or wet weather. The patient's first movements of the day are usually very painful, but the pain subsides with further movement, and warmth helps usually helps.

The skin will itch and burn with blistering spots, which seep clear fluid if scratched. Eruptions will be particularly bad on hairier parts of the body, such as in the cradle cap. The skin can also be very hot, but it is better for hot water.

Rhus tox is often indicated in shingles (page 128) and is one of the main remedies for chicken pox (page 111), where there is restlessness and a great deal of itching.

MODALITIES
Worse: *wet, cold drafts; beginning of motion; resting; sprains; over-exertion; after midnight*
Better: *continued motion; rubbing; warmth; heat; moving affected parts; stretching the limbs*

Common Uses
• Injuries • Sprains • Arthritis
• Rheumatism • Chicken pox • Shingles

Ruta

Rue grows in dry and sheltered places. It is an evergreen plant that is native to southern Europe and was originally brought to this country by the Romans. The name rue comes from the Greek word *reuo*, meaning 'to set free'. In homoeopathy it is used for injuries and sprains, restoring freedom of movement, and thus living up to its name.

FULL NAME
Ruta graveolens
(Plant family: Rutaceae)

COMMON NAME
• Rue
• Herb of grace

MAIN INDICATIONS

MENTAL AND EMOTIONAL

Ruta patients are weak and despairing. They may have a feeling of dissatisfaction and generally display fears of anything new.

PHYSICAL

Ruta is a good remedy following use of the remedy Arnica (page 28). It can be used for injury or bruising to bones, fibrous tissue, tendons, cartilage or the periosteum, which is the tissue covering the bone.

This remedy is mostly indicated when there is an injury or a sprain involving the periosteum of the wrists and ankles. The body is sore, aching and bruised, and there is a feeling of restlessness. It is an ideal remedy for treating strains around the joints and is also used for persistent stiffness after a sprain or strain. Limbs can feel heavy and weak, with pains in the hips and bones of the legs, causing unsteadiness when walking. After straining the back, the legs may feel very weak. Ruta is often given when the remedy Rhus tox (page 90) fails to work.

Ruta is a good remedy for eye complaints, especially eyestrain, which is then followed by a headache. Eyes can be red, hot and painful after reading small print or when the room is not properly lit, weakening the eye muscles.

Ruta can be used for sciatica, which is worse when the patient lies down or during the evening but gets better during the day. It is also effective for osteo-arthritis, stemming from an old sprained ankle or knee injury. It is recommended for housemaid's knee, tennis elbow and rheumatism, too, especially when these are caused by over-straining or over-exertion.

Common Uses

• Injuries • Sprains and strains • Bruises
• Eyestrain

MODALITIES

Worse: *lying or sitting down; eyestrain; wind; cold air; damp; sprains; injury from over-exertion*
Better: *warmth; rubbing; lying on the back*

91

FULL NAME
Sepia officinalis

COMMON NAMES
• Cuttlefish
• Squid

Sepia

Sepia is a dark reddish-brown pigment obtained from the inky secretion of cuttlefish, molluscs that are most commonly found in the Mediterranean, northeast Atlantic, North Sea and the English Channel. Cuttlefish come from the same family as clams, oysters, mussels and snails, the difference being that the others live within their shell, whereas the cuttlefish exposes its flesh to the outside world. There is a great deal of phosphorus contained in the cuttlefish, and its colour can change like a chameleon's. Cuttlefish are smart, despite their apparent inertia: they dart quickly towards their prey or away from their enemy, and they can moodily snap out in annoyance or provocation.

This description of this remedy's source highlights some characteristics of Sepia types. The shape of the cuttlefish bears a great resemblance to the female uterus, and we will see that Sepia has an important affinity with the female reproductive organs and the emotions that run alongside them.

MAIN INDICATIONS

MENTAL AND EMOTIONAL

Sepia relates mainly to women and female reproduction. Patients feel exhausted, run down and at the end of their tether. They work hard in every aspect of their lives but have not been particularly nourished or nurtured themselves, and so, as a result, their entire constitution often feels below par. They can no longer cope with any emotional demands and become increasingly irritable, depressed and indifferent. This is especially true when communicating with their loved ones. Like the moody cuttlefish, Sepia types will snap, fluctuating from one mood to another. They want to be all right, but they get depressed and feel that they no longer know who they are. They will cry easily – just talking makes them sob – and they don't know where the tears are coming from.

Sexuality is very important, and many symptoms arise at the time of puberty, menstruation or pregnancy. Despite the importance of sex, it is often looked upon with indifference, especially when it is demanded rather than offered. They feel incapable of love, hence the shut-down, which may lead to feelings of guilt, inadequacy and despair.

Sepia patients can feel so low that they see their unhappiness as never-ending and find it difficult to recall the last happy period in their lives.

92

This feeling, coupled with the shutting down of emotions, can lead to mental fogginess and a distracted air.

A rebelliousness is present, especially concerning female issues, and they may masculinize themselves, feeling that there is no room in this world for female sensitivity.

Sepia types nearly always feel better for being busy and active; they need stimulation to function and are often highly intelligent and perceptive. They are observant of, and sensitive to, other people's vulnerabilities but then find it difficult to express these thoughts in a constructive way.

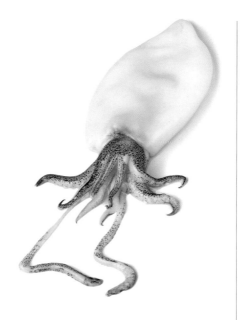

PHYSICAL

As Sepia is a predominantly female remedy, the ailments that it is used for centre on female issues. Sepia can be used very effectively in acute bouts of morning sickness during pregnancy, especially when the expectant mother is nauseous at the thought or sight of any food.

At times of menstruation the patient may have heavy, bearing-down pains in the pelvic area, and the lower back and uterus will ache, perhaps even leading to a prolapse. They find it difficult to hold on to anything, and they may even suffer urine seepage.

Muscle tone is poor and the body may start to sag; this may affect circulation, which becomes sluggish, giving rise to varicose veins, low blood pressure and constipation. The extremities of the body, such as fingers and toes, often feel the cold, although they will warm up quickly after exercise.

Due to the hormonal disturbances, habitual miscarriage is very common, making Sepia a very useful remedy after an abortion as a way of stabilizing the hormones.

Migraines can be severe, with a stinging head pain that causes nausea. The whole head becomes super-sensitized, and the face may be yellow and sallow. Herpes, thrush and ringworm are common, and during the menopause hot flushes are extreme, with offensive perspiration. Food cravings are well indicated.

Common Uses

- Exhaustion • Irritability • Menopause
- Morning sickness • Period pains

MODALITIES

Worse: *lying on left side; noise; excitement; cold; washing; eating; menstruation; menopause; too much mental stimulation; milk; fats; gentle exercise; thunderstorms; smell of food; bright lights*

Better: *warmth of the bed; hot applications; exercise; hard pressure – especially on the back; open air; cold drinks; lying on the right side*

Silica

FULL NAME
Silicea terra

SOURCE
• Silicon dioxide

Silica is found in abundance in the earth and is one of the main elements of flint, quartz and sandstone. It is one of the homoeopathic remedies naturally present in the tissues of the body, known as tissue salts.

MAIN INDICATIONS

MENTAL AND EMOTIONAL

Silica people lack stamina. There is a submissive tendency arising from insufficient energy to hold on to and defend their own point of view. They will not oppose anybody else, even if they think those people are in the wrong. They tend to be refined, intelligent, easy going, mild and reserved, although they make friends and talk about themselves easily. They are not demanding of other people's time, impatient or time-wasters when it comes to trivial matters. Feelings of sensitivity run high with these types: Silica children will take a reprimand to heart – they do not forget it and their behaviour is easily suppressed. They can also grow up with fixed ideas.

Silica is a good remedy to give for anticipatory fears – such as before exams, public speaking, and so on. The Silica person can be afraid of failure, trying to do well in whatever is undertaken, but at the same time is are easily worn out, especially by long periods of concentration. Silica types can be obstinate and irritable, trying passively to control others to cover their underlying timidity. As children, they may learn to read and write slowly and have difficulty in understanding. They lack grit and are oversensitive to noise, touch, light and criticism. They also tend to avoid confrontation whenever possible.

PHYSICAL

Silica children are thin and delicate, often with weak ankles, large heads and distended bellies. Their heads and faces tend to sweat, rather than the whole body. Any symptoms often develop in cold, damp weather, although they generally improve in cold, drier weather.

The skin may be moist and scaly and suffer from eruptions, such as acne. Silica will speed up the formation of abscesses and boils and help to eliminate foreign bodies, such as splinters, warts, pimples, pustules and suppurating cavities. It should be taken for complaints that are caused by suppressed discharges, particularly sweat. In this case, however, Silica can lead to thick, catarrhal discharges.

Headaches will also be common for Silica types, including those that feel chronic, and induce nausea and vomiting. These may start in the morning, at the back of the head, and by midday will reach the forehead. Some headaches rise from the nape of the neck and move to one eye, especially the right eye. They may occur weekly and appear to be worse at night because of factors such as light, noise, cold air and studying. Heat relieves the pain, as does pressure and wrapping the head. Profuse head sweats may accompany the headaches.

Blocked tear ducts or ulcerations on the cornea may hamper eyesight, and styes are commonplace. The ears of the Silica type can sometimes exude an offensive thick yellow discharge in association with middle-ear infections and catarrh of the Eustachian tube, which can lead to temporary deafness. The nose may become affected by hard, crusty scabs, catarrh, and there may be a loss of taste and smell.

This is the remedy to use when teeth tend to break and crumble. The enamel will start to come away, and mouth abscesses will form in the gums, which will improve, however, with warmth. Enlarged tonsils and chronic sore throats with enlarged glands will also benefit when Silica is taken.

Problems of the stomach include hiccups, nausea and vomiting, with an aversion to warm food. There is a dislike of meat, and milk will aggravate the symptoms. Patients have a preference for cold things, such as ice cream and iced water. Constipation is caused by inactivity of the rectum, the stool being partly expelled only to then recede. In women this tends to be worse before and during periods.

Other women's complaints include cysts in the vagina, fistula openings and abscesses along the vulva, healing to leave hard nodules. Silica is distinguished by offensive-smelling, bloody discharges during periods, which can start simply from excitement or when breast-feeding. There can be profuse milky leucorrhoea and hard lumps in the breasts. There may also be breast abscesses and a tendency to experience difficulties during pregnancy, perhaps even miscarrying.

Silica types' coughs are dry and tickly with hoarseness, becoming worse when cold and better for warm drinks. During the day they may expectorate green mucus, and colds will go to the chest. Silica can be a good remedy for asthma, bronchitis and the later stages of pneumonia.

Common Uses

- Abscesses • Boils • Catarrh • Coughs
- Colds • Headaches • Earache
- Mouth ulcers • Splinters

MODALITIES

Worse: *cold; noise; draughts; light; damp; pressure; mental exertion; full moon; alcohol; nervous excitement*

Better: *warmth; wrapping up the head; summer; wet, humid weather; profuse urination*

FULL NAME
Spongia tosta

SOURCE
• Toasted sea
  sponge

Spongia

Sea sponges found in the Mediterranean are used to make this remedy. They are lightly toasted and then ground to a powder.

MAIN INDICATIONS

MENTAL AND EMOTIONAL

There is a lot of fear and anxiety within the picture of this remedy. Spongia types fear that they are going to die and will often wake from sleep in terror. This remedy is very similar to the remedy Aconite (page 20), although the Aconite patient usually displays more fear. It is important to compare the two before diagnosing one of them.

PHYSICAL

It is mainly the respiratory centre that is affected in the picture of this remedy. It is good for coughs that take several days to develop and when there is inflammation and a dry, rough sensation in the throat, with dryness in the nasal passages too, which inevitably gives rise to sneezing. It may develop into a dry, hoarse cough, which can sound like a dog barking.

Spongia is a good remedy to give children with croup. Young patients can have a suffocating cough, which will wake them up, and they will be fearful, anxious and tearful. The cough tends to be tight, hollow, barking or crowing and gets worse after midnight. If the remedy Aconite is given for the cough earlier in the evening and there is temporary improvement but it recurs in the early hours, then try Spongia. If the cough returns at around 5 p.m., or the next day, try Hepar sulph (page 60).

The remedy Spongia is excellent to use when breathing sounds and feels as if it is through a sponge. There can be burning in the throat, which gets worse at night. It is also a useful remedy for asthma where there is a lot of wheezing and whistling; the asthma attack can be relieved by sitting up and bending forwards. The element of dryness is an important keynote: Spongia is a good remedy to use for dry coughs that get worse on successive nights. Mucus can develop after several days, with a feeling of fullness in the chest and expectoration is usually easy.

MODALITIES

Worse: *sore throat symptoms, which get worse from eating; sweet things; warm drinks*

Better: *lying with the head low; bending forwards*

Common Uses
• Cough • Croup • Asthma

Staphysagria

Staphysagria is an ancient remedy from a bluish-purple biennial plant that was utilized as a medicine as long ago as the time of Hippocrates, initially for promoting vomiting. The kernels were mainly used, although thought to be very dangerous, because they could cause choking and strangulation; the seeds are also extremely hot and spicy. It is these kernels, or seeds, that are used in the preparation of the homoeopathic remedy.

This remedy has a strong affinity with the nervous system, which can become so sensitized that it can lead to paralysis, slowness of the pulse and eventual death.

FULL NAME
Delphinium staphysagria
(Plant family: Ranunculaceae)

COMMON NAME
• Palmated larkspur

MAIN INDICATIONS

MENTAL AND EMOTIONAL

The gentle and sweet Staphysagria picture, like that of Nat mur (page 76), is, sadly, characterized by the theme of suppressed emotions, mostly due to romantic relationships and grief. Patients can be incredibly excitable and easily aroused, and yet they have great difficulty in displaying this, allowing themselves to feel powerless, resigned and passive. Patients can also over-romanticize everyday situations in great detail, becoming easily disappointed with any emotional failures they encounter. They have strong sexual desires, yet find them difficult to communicate.

The rudeness of others is a mortifying experience to Staphysagria types and they can easily take offence and feel humiliated; once again, this is internalized. The suppression of the emotional state can lead to an inflexibility on the mental sphere, and forgetfulness can prevail, along with mental inertia and possible dementia.

PHYSICAL

The nervous system is strongly affected with extreme sensitivity to light, noise and touch. Cystitis is very common, with a constant urge to urinate, especially when there is a new sexual partner. Staphysagria is also an excellent remedy for use after surgical operations.

Recurrent styes occur and warts are commonly seen. The homoeopathic tincture is often used as a hair lotion to prevent head lice.

Common Uses
• Cystitis • Head lice • Styes

MODALITIES

Worse: *emotions; humiliation; sexual excesses; cold drinks; lacerations; night; morning; tobacco; touch*

Better: *warmth; rest; breakfast*

FULL NAME

Sulphur, the element

COMMON NAME

• Brimstone

Sulphur

S ulphur is a well-known substance – from volcanoes and stink bombs to bathing in sulphur pools, we have all had some experience of this element. Sulphur is a substance that when burned, produces a vapour that re-condenses to form a yellowish, crystalline powder. It doesn't evaporate and disappear, unlike Phosphorus (page 84), but stays very much earth-bound.

Its main medicinal uses have been concentrated around ailments of the skin, particularly as the main ingredient of Epsom salts and intensively in medicinal spas. As a homoeopathic remedy, we see a continuation of this affinity with our skin.

Sulphur has an impressive picture in terms of the number of symptoms that are listed in homoeopathic books. Because of its huge scope, this remedy is difficult to capture in a few paragraphs, and only a brief outline of Sulphur's main characteristics can be given here.

MAIN INDICATIONS

MENTAL AND EMOTIONAL

The strength and inflation of the ego plays a very big part in this picture, with the phrase 'me, myself and I' lurking behind most actions. Sulphur types can be selfish, censorious, thoughtless and unconcerned for others. Their minds are full of ideas and theories, in which they have enormous belief, and they take very unkindly to being told otherwise. They love to spread their immense knowledge in a philosophical way, and their imagination can be incredibly expansive. The problem, however, is that their heads are often in the clouds, and, despite their philosophical thinking, they never get to the root of anything. It is as if they just don't have enough time, or inclination, to finish the job. The ideas can be so prolific that they are just unable to cope, so an intense laziness can set in instead. Despite their belief in their own genius, this lack of persistence will let them down. The practical side of Sulphur types is also flawed by the lack of final execution.

The Sulphur character loves a good argument – just for the sake of it – and will have no qualms about telling people how to live their lives; these people love to be the centre of attention. Their tempers can be explosive, like volcanoes. They will be quick to defend any criticisms and are somewhat unforgiving towards those who criticize their behaviour.

Sulphur types can be incredibly messy, and, like the 'bag lady' in the street, they generally think that any old rags can look beautiful – another extension of their imagination. One may find a polarity in their character whereby they are very tidy at work and yet their home is a picture of chaos. If they do create any order in the home, things will look immaculate until a cupboard is opened and everything that has been stuffed in there comes tumbling out!

The constant influx of ideas and thoughts can induce a great amount of worrying, even hypochondria. Sulphur types are often referred to as the constitutional grumblers.

PHYSICAL

On the physical level, Sulphur has a very hot-blooded picture, and the whole circulatory system can emit flushes of local heat to various different parts of the body. The heat is burning and throbbing, causing any affected parts to look incredibly red. The feet can feel so hot that covering them up, with clothing or bed linen, is unbearable. All the orifices will burn with pain – the ears, eyes, nostrils, mouth and, in particular, the anus.

These types can look very dirty and unclean, and are sometimes known as 'the great unwashed'. Body odour may present problems, as Sulphur patients can smell fairly offensive. They are often full of gas, producing exceptionally smelly flatulence.

The skin is scaly, with a great deal of itchy, burning rashes and various eruptions that are particularly acute along the hairline. Scratching these areas feels blissful at first but is followed by a burning, smarting pain. The skin symptoms are worse for heat: from washing with warm water to the heat of the bed or woollen clothing. The skin can easily become infected and ulcerated, and many of the complaints alternate with other ailments, especially asthma.

The stomach rumbles, and there may be a great urge to get out of bed at around 5 a.m. to go to the toilet; all the symptoms are worse between 2 and 5 a.m. Extreme hunger sets in at about 11 a.m., when there is a desire for something to snack on.

Sulphur is a particularly good remedy for haemorrhoids that feel sore and raw and that are burning, smarting and bleed easily.

Patients will often hold their bodies in stooped positions, or, alternatively, they will be hunched up in a chair. Finally, there is a great love of alcohol, spices, sweets, fat and beer.

Common Uses
• Diarrhoea • Gastroenteritis • Eczema
• Haemorrhoids

MODALITIES

Worse: *taking a hot bath; becoming too hot; washing; early morning; at 11 a.m.*

Better: *open air; moving about; dry heat; warm applications; warm drinks; sweating*

Thuja

*T*huja occidentalis* is an evergreen conifer, found in the damp regions of North America. It can grow to 45 foot (14 m) in height and is thought to have a more elegant appearance than that of its relative, the red western cedar. It grows very slowly, with a twisted, gnarled trunk and is covered with regimented cones and flat scales. The wood has a sweet scent and is highly resistant to decay.

Thuja occidentalis is often used for sturdy outdoor structures such as fence poles and tiles and the tree itself is sometimes used in gardens to provide privacy. There is a link between the tree's outdoor use and the acutely secretive, hidden nature of Thuja in its homoeopathic form.

The remedy is prepared from the fresh green twigs, and it is a substance that affects the concentration of salt, water and electrolytes in the body.

MAIN INDICATIONS

MENTAL AND EMOTIONAL

There is a great sense of being closed and hidden within this picture. Thuja types do not like to reveal anything, preferring instead to keep their ideas and emotions close to their chests, thus reflecting the use of the Thuja tree to make things private or keep them hidden. Somehow, they mask their symptoms by a well-manufactured image that has been tried and tested on more than one occasion. Thuja characters are known as the 'great masqueraders', and they can easily interpret what is expected of them within certain situations and perform accordingly; they are the true chameleons of society.

It is important to understand why they need to do this, and just as Thuja trees are grown to hide the gardens that lie behind them, we need to look at the emotions being hidden. Internally, there is great fragility, with a strong sensation that the body is as vulnerable as glass. There is a strong feeling of being unlovable, and this very low self-esteem encourages Thuja types to conceal what they feel is their true nature, in order to be liked. This negative image may stem from childhood experiences of being told they were not good enough. They produce what they believe to be an acceptable version of themselves: inside they perceive themselves to be ugly and deceitful, and an observer can sometimes sense this. They can be manipulative and harsh in an attempt to avoid real emotional contact with people – something that fills them with fear – in case others find something they don't want to be seen. The Thuja person is extremely controlled.

The concept of fixed ideas is also strong with Thuja, and there may be a tendency for fanaticism, either religious or delusionary, concerning the body. This may lead to anorexia or indeed other products of obsession about bodily appearance.

PHYSICAL

The discharges in the Thuja types are often green or yellowy-green, and the symptoms are always much worse in cold, wet weather. The face may seem waxy, shiny and almost translucent, as if smeared with grease – again prompting us to think of a mask. In fact, all of the skin can be quite oily, with a sweetish smell, like the sweetness of the tree. This is a remedy renowned for external growths, with warts, condylamata and polyps often being among the chief complaints.

The body can feel very frail, and sometimes the abdomen may feel uncomfortable, making patients feel as if there is something alive inside them. Perhaps this is a reflection of the inner self they are trying to conceal. The abdomen can become distended with uncomfortable wind. There is a great desire for chocolate, cold food and drink and a peculiar desire for raw onions.

Nails can be problematic, becoming soft, ribbed or brittle. They may easily

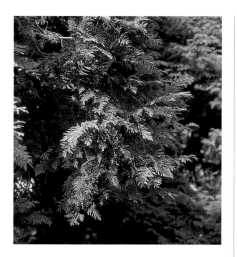

crack and crumble, causing them to look very distorted. There may also be a strange sensation of painful soles of the feet. Sudden numbness or paralysis can affect the limbs, making them feel completely dead.

The Thuja headache can feel as if a nail is being driven in, and there can be a painful pressure at the root of the nose.

Being unwell after vaccination is also a keynote in Thuja patients, perhaps mirroring their hatred of intrusion.

Thuja is a difficult remedy to use at home, despite being readily available at chemists, and is usually prescribed as a constitutional remedy by a qualified homoeopath. The homoeopathic tincture, however, is often used in a diluted form for warts and verrucae.

All symptoms of this remedy tend to be much worse at either 3 a.m. or 3 p.m.

Common Uses

• Warts • After vaccination

MODALITIES

Worse: *talking; overheating; cold; damp; 3 a.m. or 3 p.m.; vaccination; tea; onions; moving around*

Better: *open air; being warm; lying on the affected side; lying on the back*

Urtica

Stinging nettles grow profusely, thriving particularly in soils that are rich in nitrogen. The poison contained in the plant is ammonium bicarbonate, which is destroyed by heat, thus making it safe to consume as a tea or soup. The strength of the nettle fibre encouraged its use in the textile industry in the seventeenth century.

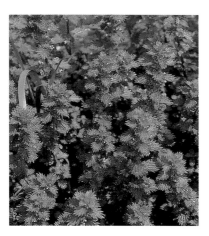

Many people are familiar with the stinging nettle, which causes irritation and inflammation at the slightest touch, although there is surprisingly little effect when the plant is grasped tightly. The dock leaf is a well-known antidote to nettle stings, although nettle juice itself will ease the skin irritation just as effectively. This gives an idea of how the nettle is used homoeopathically. In herbal spheres, Urtica has been used for centuries and is a renowned blood cleanser, containing high levels of vitamin C and iron.

MAIN INDICATIONS

MENTAL AND EMOTIONAL

As with the remedy Euphrasia (page 54), Urtica has no particular mental or emotional symptoms; it is used solely to treat physical complaints.

PHYSICAL

Urtica is best known for its effect on minor first-degree burns when the pain is intensely stinging and itchy. As well as being available in tablet form, this remedy can be applied to burns in the form of a tincture, diluted into a cup of cool, boiled water. The resulting solution is then soaked into a piece of gauze and applied to the affected area, keeping the gauze moist until a scab appears. Urtica will quickly relieve the pain and help heal the burn with minimum scarring.

This remedy can also relieve the skin rash urticaria, which covers the whole body with red, itchy blotches and is often related to food allergies. The rash feels much worse if the person is too warm, such as after a hot bath. Lying down in a cool room will help to relieve the symptoms. The nature of the stinging pain makes this a good remedy for insect bites, including bee and wasp stings, and burning pains such as cystitis.

Common Uses
• Burns • Insect bites • Stings • Urticaria

Veratrum alb

FULL NAME
Veratrum album
(Plant family:
Liliaceae)

COMMON NAME
• White hellebore

Veratrum album, meaning 'white truth', grows high in the mountains of the Swiss Alps, where it thrives in this elevated position. The root is used in the preparation of the remedy. However, in the past, the poison from this plant was used on the tips of arrows and daggers with fatal consequences. When eaten in its raw state the plant produces unpleasant burning pains, which are accompanied by severe vomiting and diarrhoea, a lowering of blood pressure and cold sweat. Many of these symptoms are seen in the remedy picture, as it is effective in severe digestive upsets.

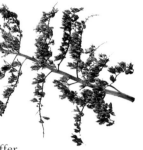

MAIN INDICATIONS

MENTAL AND EMOTIONAL

Veratrum is associated with people who are proud – people who can be very patronizing and arrogant. Their social position is important to them, and they work hard to get to the top, even if deceit is needed. They are inclined to be subservient to those above them – those with status – but unpleasant to those below. They suffer greatly if their pride has been hurt, especially if it involves rejection, and have a need to stand out from the crowd. They may adopt a strong religious stance, appearing to be overly pure and evangelical.

PHYSICAL

This remedy mainly centres around the digestive system, coming into its own for chronic diarrhoea, when the patient has collapsed quite suddenly. Patients feel icy cold, with a cold sweat, and may have the sensation that cold water runs through their veins. Despite the coldness, they like to suck ice cubes and eat cold food. They can appear blue and have cold breath, as with the remedy Carbo Veg (page 43). They can suffer intense nausea, with sharp cramping pains. Stools will be watery and green and may simultaneously occur with vomiting, diarrhoea, dizziness and fainting.

Veratrum is a useful remedy for intensely painful, cramping periods, which may come early and be heavy. Again, nausea, vomiting, diarrhoea and fainting accompany the pain.

Patients may also desire acidic foods and drink, especially craving fruit, although this will inevitably contribute to their feeling of discomfort.

Common Uses
• Nausea • Diarrhoea • Gastroenteritis
• Period pains

MODALITIES

Worse: *hot food; fruit; change of season; injured pride*
Better: *cold food; being warm; hot drinks*

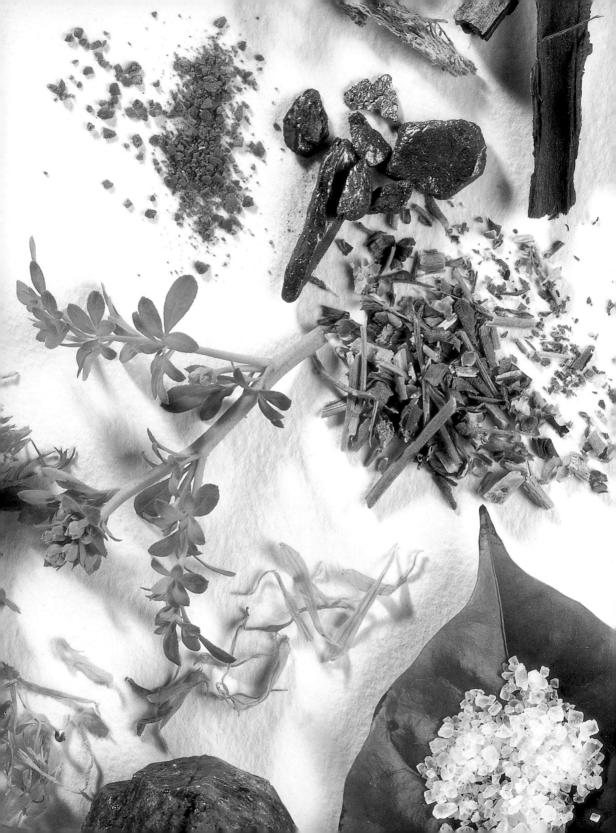

Ailments &
Remedies

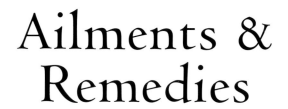

This section sets out in a simple repertory
index the conditions and situations that
may be helped by the homoeopathic remedies
described in the Materia Medica. Each ailment is
described briefly, and then the remedies appropriate
for treatment are listed below, in many cases
allowing an initial choice to be made. The chosen
remedy can then be explored and confirmed in more
detail in the Materia Medica section. Suggested
dosages are also given.

It is important to seek professional advice, from
either your homoeopath or medical practitioner,
especially if symptoms are chronic or severe, or if
they persist or even if it seems appropriate.

Abscess

An abscess is a local collection of pus that may become inflamed, causing throbbing pain, heat and redness. Take the remedy in the 6c potency three times a day for 2–3 days but stop on improvement.

Apis – *stinging, burning pains; abscess is hot, swollen and painful when touched*

Belladonna – *throbbing, burning pains; abscess is red, inflamed and painful when touched*

Hepar sulph – *stitching, splinter-like pains; pus is forming and the area feels sore and tender*

Silica – *pus has formed and the abscess is draining slowly; discharge is offensive; remedy will speed up the draining process*

Accidents

These remedies will help in a first-aid situation for minor incidents, but you should always seek professional advice if there is unconsciousness or profuse haemorrhaging. Bach's Rescue Remedy (see Glossary – page 134) can also be useful for shock following an accident. Also, diluted Hypericum and Calendula tincture applied externally can soothe minor cuts and grazes. Take the remedy in 6c potency three times a day for 2–3 days, or 3–4 doses in 30c every four hours.

Arnica – *the first remedy to give after an accident; will help with shock, bruising and any haemorrhaging that is present*

Aconite – *for any initial shock or fear*

Hypericum – *for accidents involving the nerves or lacerated wounds with shooting pains*

Acne

This skin condition is due to over-activity of the oil-producing glands arising from hormonal changes. Spots, pustules and blackheads appear on the skin and may become infected. Acne is most commonly found among teenagers and women at the time of their periods. Use the remedy in 6c potency three times a day for ten days.

Calc phos – *acne in teenagers; skin is pale and sweaty*

Sulphur – *skin looks generally unhealthy*

Silica – *helps with elimination when spots are slow to clear; skin can be sweaty*

Allergies

Allergies occur as the result of an over-reaction between antigens and antibodies within the body. There can be many causes, including genetic inheritance. It will be helpful to see a professional practitioner for constitutional treatment if an allergic response is common. Take the remedies in the 6c potency three times a day for 1–2 days.

Apis – *skin looks swollen or puffy and feels hot, with fiery, stinging pains*

Ferrum phos – *helps reduce the first signs
of inflammation*
Rhus tox – *skin is blistered and itchy;
worse on hairier parts of the body*
Urtica – *skin allergies that are intensely
itchy; skin looks red and blotchy (this is
often a food-related allergy)*

Anaemia

Anaemia occurs when the blood does
not carry enough oxygen due to a
lack of red blood cells or changes in
the levels of haemoglobin. Iron is
essential for the formation of red
blood cells, so if it is lacking in your
diet or there is a persistent loss of
blood, anaemia can occur. Take the
remedy in 6x potency three times a
day for ten days.
Ferrum phos – *this is one of the tissue salts
that enables the body to absorb iron
more efficiently*

Anxiety

Anxiety produces feelings of unease
and apprehension and maifests itself
physically through heart palpitations,
sweating and diarrhoea. Take the
remedies in the 6c potency three
times a day for 1–2 days. If there is
prolonged anxiety then it is advisable
to talk to a professional practitioner.
Arg nit – *anticipatory anxiety with
diarrhoea; the 'what if?' scenario;
fear of flying*

Arsenicum – *anxiety, with extreme
restlessness, particularly concerning health*
Gelsemium – *anxiety before an exam;
patient may feel paralysed by fear*
Kali phos – *anxiety from nervous
exhaustion and sleeplessness*
Lycopodium – *anxiety before an event but
better once it has begun; lack of confidence*
Ignatia – *anxiety from grief; may become
hysterical and faint*

Arthritis

Arthritis is a painful condition in
which joints swell due to cartilage or
synovial inflammation. It is important
to see a professional practitioner for
treatment of this condition; however,
the remedies below may bring short-
term relief. Take the 6c potency three
times a day for 2–3 weeks or less if
the symptoms improve.
Arnica – *arthritis as the result of an
injury; feels bruised and sore*
Bryonia – *any movement makes the joint
more painful; hard pressure helps to
relieve the pain*
Ferrum phos – *sudden inflammation of the
joint; good for the initial stages*
Ledum – *stiff, burning pains in the joint;
cold compresses ease the pain*
Rhus tox – *joints feel stiff and painful
when first moved but get better with
further movement*
Ruta – *joints feel stiff and sore; movement
makes the pain worse*

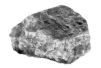

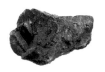

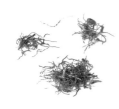

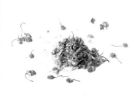

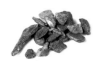

Asthma

Asthma is a serious respiratory condition that needs to be treated by a professional practitioner. The remedies below are to be used in acute situations to help relieve spasms. Take the remedy in the 6c potency every hour for four hours.

Arsenicum – *great restlessness and prostration; prop up head with pillow; worse after midnight*

Carbo veg – *feelings of suffocation, combined with a desire to be fanned; patient looks pale or may turn blue during an attack; weakness prevails*

Drosera – *cough comes in fits and starts; chest must be held during an attack; unable to get enough air and may be aggravated by heat*

Kali carb – *must bring the elbows down to the knees during an attack; worse between 2 and 5 a.m.*

Mag phos – *will help to relax any spasms*

Nat sulph – *attack is triggered by dampness; must sit up and hold chest during an attack; worse between 4 and 5 a.m.*

Backache

Many things cause back pain, and it is, therefore, always important to know the cause before treatment. Manipulation by an osteopath or chiropractor, for example, is advisable if appropriate. Take the remedy in a 6c potency three times a day for 2–3 days, or three doses of 30c eight hours apart.

Arnica – *back feels bruised; aches after an accident, injury or from over-exertion*

Bellis perennis – *pain in the coccyx after a fall*

Hypericum – *spinal injuries that involve the nerves; shooting nerve pain up or down the back*

Kali carb – *lower back pain with shooting pains down the legs; back pain during labour*

Mag phos – *cramping, spasmodic nerve pains felt in the back, relieved by warmth and massage*

Rhus tox – *stiffness and muscular tension from over-straining or injury; worse when first moving and also when damp*

Bites and stings

Some people react severely to bites and stings, with painful swellings and, in some cases, breathing difficulties. It is always best to seek professional advice if you are unsure of any reaction. Take the remedy in the 6c potency three times a day for 2–3 days, or one tablet of 30c every four hours, stopping on improvement.

Apis – *wasp and bee stings with burning, stinging pains; skin will be hot, puffy and inflamed with redness; may feel worse with hot applications*

Hypericum – *punctured skin with shooting, darting pains that move away from the injury site; skin is inflamed and hot*

Ledum – *puncture wounds and bites; skin is sensitive to touch; skin looks puffy and red but feels cold; will generally be better for any cold applications*

Boils

Boils occur due to inflammation at the root of hair follicles, causing red, painful swelling. In order to avoid infection, bathe the boil in diluted Hypericum and Calendula tincture (see Introduction – page 14), for example. Take the remedy in the 6c potency three times a day for five days.

Belladonna – *hot, throbbing painful boils; skin is sensitive to the touch*

Silica – *boils that have started to suppurate and are slow to heal; offensive discharges*

Breast-feeding

Breast-feeding is a particular time of bonding for mother and baby but it can be distressing if problems arise. Seek professional advice if symptoms persist or you feel worried in any way. Homoeopathic remedies can also be used to help increase or decrease breast milk flow, or to stop it all together once breast-feeding is no longer required. Take the remedy in the 6c potency three times a day for five days.

China – *exhaustion and weakness from fluid loss*

Kali phos – *exhaustion and debility from loss of sleep; a good nerve restorative*

Phytolacca – *hard, painful breasts with spasms of pain during feeding; cracked and sore nipples*

Silica – *threatened abscess on the nipple, reducing breast milk flow*

Bronchitis

In acute bronchitis there is inflammation and infection of the respiratory tract, causing breathing difficulties with painful coughing and possible fever. Take the remedy in the 6c potency three times a day for 2–3 days, or in 30c for three doses eight hours apart. Chronic bronchitis, however, must be treated by a professional practitioner.

Aconite – *cough that comes suddenly after exposure to cold, dry winds; short, dry cough that is worse at night; fearful*

Ant tart – *cough sounds rattling; patient is unable to expel any mucus, giving the sensation of drowning; weakness and exhaustion prevail*

Arsenicum – *anxiety and restlessness; suffocative cough with a thirst for small sips of water*

Bryonia – *hard, dry, barking cough; must hold the chest when coughing due to pain; irritable with desire to be left alone*

Causticum – *dry, hollow cough with pain in the chest; throat feels raw; may urinate while coughing*

Drosera – *dry, suffocative, barking cough; may feel the need for company, especially on waking at night*

Ferrum phos – *first signs of the cough with fever and inflammation*

Hepar sulph – *dry, croupy cough that has been present for a long time; the patient is chilly and irritable*

Ipecac – *dry, hacking, suffocative cough that may be followed by vomiting to raise the mucus; nausea; desire for fresh air*

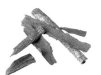

Kali carb – *dry, hacking cough that sounds like a smoker's cough; weakness and exhaustion prevail*

Phosphorus – *burning sensation in the lungs; tight, hard cough; fearful and exhausted*

Spongia – *barking, hollow cough; dry and burning throat; chest feels tight; may be fearful*

Bruises

Bruises are usually caused by a blow or a fall, causing blood vessels to leak and the blood then clots beneath the skin. Take the remedy in the 6c potency three times a day for 1–2 days.

Arnica – *first major remedy commonly used when treating bruises after injuries and accidents*

Bellis perennis – *deep internal bruising after surgery; abdominal bruising in pregnancy from the baby kicking*

Burns

Minor burns can be treated at home, but more serious ones, where all layers of the skin have been significantly damaged, must have immediate medical attention. The following remedies will help with any shock or pain that a patient may suffer. Take the remedy in the 6c potency three times a day for 2–3 days.

Cantharis – *burns and scolds where the skin has blistered; raw, stinging pains*

Causticum – *serious burns that are raw and extremely painful*

Urtica – *minor burns that are stinging, painful and itchy*

Catarrh

Increased production of mucus and irritation and inflammation of the mucous membranes are the symptoms of this complaint. If you have chronic catarrh it is better to be treated constitutionally by your homoeopath. Dairy products can often increase mucus production, and you may wish to reduce your dairy intake for a period of time. Take the 6c potency three times a day until symptoms improve.

Calc fluor – *long-term catarrh that is yellowish-green in colour*

Hepar sulph – *thick, yellow catarrh that smells foul; worse in cold, dry winds*

Kali bich – *stuffed-up sensation at the root of the nose; thick, stringy catarrh that comes out in gluey ropes*

Kali carb – *thick, yellow catarrh that is crusty in the morning on waking; head feels congested*

Nat mur – *watery, bland discharge from the nose*

Pulsatilla – *thick yellow, green or white bland discharge; profuse during the day, blocked up at night; will improve with fresh air*

Silica – *thick, yellow catarrh that can form into crusty scabs in the nose; loss of taste and smell*

Chicken pox

Chicken pox is highly contagious around 24 hours before the itchy, blister-like rash appears, generally first on the back or stomach. It continues to be infectious until scabs form. If these scabs are scratched, scars will appear. It is important, therefore, to obtain relief from the itchiness as much as possible. The spots are very itchy, and a fever is usually present. Although this ailment is usually associated with young children, adults are not immune and may contract it in the form of shingles. The remedies below may help to ease the pain and discomfort of the blisters and scabs. Take the remedy in the 6c potency three times a day until the symptoms improve.

Ant tart – *slow-developing rash; exhaustion and lethargy prevail; child is irritable but still wants to be held for comfort; rattling cough may accompany the rash*

Arsenicum – *restlessness, with a desire to scratch until the eruptions bleed; burning pains; child chilly and thirsty for small sips of water*

Belladonna – *hot, flushed face with fever and dilated pupils; the child may start to hallucinate*

Pulsatilla – *tearful child, needing lots of cuddles; feverish but thirstless, with a desire for fresh air*

Rhus tox – *intolerable itching and burning; eruptions that make the child restless; better in warmer conditions*

Chilblains

Chilblains are essentially a circulatory problem, mainly occurring in the fingers and toes, where the blood vessels start to itch and burn. Ideally, steps should be made to improve circulation in the long term. However, in the short term, to help with the pain, take the remedy in the 6x potency three times a day for ten days.

Calc fluor – *chilblains are badly cracked and chapped; this is a good remedy for improving circulation*

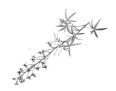

Colds

It is thought that we all need a cold now and again to eliminate toxicity from our bodies. Colds are the result of inflammation in the mucous membranes of the nose and throat. These remedies will aid the speeding up of this detoxifying process rather than suppressing the cold, as more typical aids may do. Take the remedy in the 6c potency three times a day for 2–3 days, or 30c every eight hours for 3–4 doses.

Aconite – *the cold starts suddenly after exposure to cold, dry winds or after a shock; sore throat, fever and headache*

Allium cepa – *sneezing, together with corrosive discharge from the nose; bland tears from the eyes; may be worse at night when the patient is over-heated; larynx starts to feel as if it is tearing*

Arsenicum – fluent discharge that makes the nose sore; lots of sneezing; patient feels restless and chilly

Eupatorium – copious catarrh with sneezing; bones feel brittle; shivering and restless

Euphrasia – eyes are watery and burning; fluid discharge from the nose during the day; stuffed up at night; chilly, yet desires fresh air

Ferrum phos – beginning stages of a cold with inflammation of the throat

Gelsemium – exhausted, weak and shivery; limbs and eyes feel heavy; throbbing headache; lack of thirst

Colic

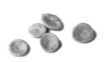

Colic is an uncomfortable, spasmodic pain in the abdomen, which is common in babies, although it can also affect adults. It may occur due to an obstruction or from certain foods, particularly those that are rich or acidic. It is best to seek advice from your homoeopath if the symptoms persist. Take the remedy in the 6c potency three times a day, stopping on improvement.

Chamomilla – irritable, restless and angry due to the pain; diarrhoea, with a sweaty head and feet

Colocynth – restlessness; cramping, twisting pain; patient must bend double and apply heat to relieve the pain; feels better when hard pressure is applied

Mag phos – severe cramping pains relieved by heat, bending double and gentle massage

Conjunctivitis

The eyes are red, swollen, painful and inflamed with this condition and there is usually a thick, bland discharge. Seek professional advice if the symptoms persist. Take the remedy in the 6c potency three times a day until symptoms improve.

Apis – stinging, burning pains; eyelids are hot, puffy and swollen

Cantharis – burning pains; red eyes; tears feel scorching

Belladonna – eyes will throb; redness and inflammation

Euphrasia – eyes feel itchy, with burning pains; swollen eyelids with possible blood-shot eyes; oozing pus

Pulsatilla – yellow-green discharge; desire for fresh air

Constipation

Constipation involves irregular bowel movements and stools that are difficult to discharge from the body. Many things can cause constipation but dietary advice is always recommended. See your homoeopath if symptoms persist. Take the remedy in the 6c potency three times a day for 2–3 days, or 30c eight hours apart for three doses.

Bryonia – hard, dry, knotty stools; thirsty

Graphites – large, knotty stools with stringy mucus; anal fissures; hungry; cold

Nux vomica – great urge for a stool; sensation as if the stool is unfinished; toxic headache

Opium – *inactive rectum; stools discharged in little, black balls; constipation occurs from shock*

Sepia – *constipation due to sluggish circulation; sensation as if there is a lump in the rectum*

Convalescence

It is always important to give yourself time to recuperate after illness. Our lifestyles often don't allow much time for this. These remedies may aid in your recovery. Take one in the 6c potency three times a day for 3–4 days, but for Calc phos and Kali phos use the 6x potency for ten days.

Calc phos – *helps with assimilation of nutrients*

Carbo veg – *exhausted and wiped out following a long illness*

China – *exhaustion after loss of bodily fluids*

Kali phos – *muscular weakness and exhaustion*

Phos ac – *emotional exhaustion or weakness after a long illness*

Corns

Corns – dead tissue in the outer layer of the skin – are often the result of poorly fitting shoes or bad posture. Addressing both these causes will help. Take the remedy in the 6x potency three times a day for ten days.

Calc fluor – *skin is hard and calloused*

Cough

Coughs differ enormously, so check the appropriate remedies in the Materia Medica for a clear differentiation. Seek professional advice if the cough persists. Take the remedy in the 6c potency three times a day for 2–3 days.

Ant tart – *rattling, bubbling cough; unable to raise the mucus; sensation as if drowning in the mucus; may end in vomiting; pale and exhausted*

Causticum – *dry, hollow cough; mucus slips down the throat; may pass urine on coughing*

Bryonia – *hard, dry cough; sticking pains in the chest aggravated by movement; must hold the chest when coughing; thirsty*

Hepar sulph – *dry, croupy cough*

Ipecac – *suffocative, rattling, wheezing cough that comes on suddenly; lungs will be full of mucus*

Phosphorus – *chest feels tight as if it is under heavy pressure; burning pains; blood-streaked sputum*

Cramp

Cramp is a painful, spasmodic, muscular contraction. Take the remedy in either the 6c or 30c potency when the cramp occurs.

Arnica – *parts feel bruised and sore; cramp after over-exertion*

Mag phos – *cramps can appear anywhere; especially good for menstrual cramps; better with warmth and rubbing*

Croup

Caution must be taken with this harsh coughing condition; professional advice should be sought if the symptoms persist. Take the remedy in the 30c potency for 1–2 doses, as required.

Aconite – *sudden onset, brought on by cold, dry winds; worse at midnight*

Hepar sulph – *suffocative cough; rattling in the chest; worse before midnight*

Spongia – *tight, hollow, barking cough; worse after midnight*

Cystitis

Cystitis is a bacterial infection of the urinary tract, bringing about the need to urinate constantly, even when the patient has only just finished urinating. When passing urine, the patient experiences a great deal of pain. It is important to stop infection moving up to the kidneys; seeking professional medical advice, therefore, is important, especially if symptoms persist or back pain is experienced. Drinking large quantities of water will help to clear the infection. Any remedy should be taken in the 6c potency three times a day for 2–3 days.

Apis – *last few drops sting and smart; frequent urge to urinate; general feelings of not being thirsty*

Cantharis – *violent burning and cutting pains when urinating; urine feels scalding*

Staphysagria – *after sex with a new partner*

Dental treatment

Regular visits to the dentist are obviously important for maintaining healthy teeth and gums, no matter what age you are, but they can be painful experiences. Use the remedies below to help the healing process and calm any feelings of anxiety. Arnica can be taken beforehand to anticipate any bruising. Take the remedy in the 30c potency in 3–4 doses, as necessary.

Arnica – *for bruising, shock and haemorrhaging; will help the healing process*

Hypericum – *shooting nerve pain following dental treatment*

Depression

It is important to seek professional advice, either from a homoeopath or a counsellor, if you are feeling depressed, and constitutional treatment is strongly advised. Refer to the Useful Addresses section (page 138) for help in locating a homoeopath in your area. You may try the following in the 30c potency, two doses eight hours apart, before seeking professional advice.

Aurum – *feelings of failure and guilt; deep, dark depression; no joy left*

Nat mur – *depression from disappointment concerning love; grief and hurt*

Phos ac – *depression from exhaustion or from caring for others*

Diarrhoea

Diarrhoea has many causes, such as food poisoning. It is vital to drink plenty of liquids to keep well hydrated and to aim to eat light, lean foods in order to starve any bacteria of fat. If the diarrhoea continues for more than 24 hours seek professional advice, or sooner in young children because dehydration can occur at a much quicker pace. Take the remedy in the 6c potency three times a day for 2–3 days, or 30c for three doses eight hours apart.

Arg nit – *diarrhoea from anxiety; spluttery; green stools with offensive smell; may be worse after eating*

Arsenicum – *burning, watery diarrhoea that comes in small amounts with prostration and restlessness; possibly caused by food poisoning; thirst for small sips of water*

Chamomilla – *especially for diarrhoea in children; looks like chopped spinach and eggs; irritability and pain*

China – *diarrhoea from eating too much fruit; copious but painless; exhaustion after defecating*

Colocynth – *food poisoning; white, jelly-like diarrhoea with cramping pains*

Merc sol – *offensive, watery diarrhoea; unpleasant smell; worse at night*

Podophyllum – *explosive, spluttery diarrhoea like rice water; painless; smells foul*

Pulsatilla – *diarrhoea from eating rich foods; may feel bloated; desire for fresh air; weepy*

Veratrum alb – *watery green stools; collapsed state; icy cold, with cold sweat; may vomit at the same time*

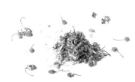

Earache

Infections in any of the tubes connecting the nose and throat are usually the cause of earache. If earaches reoccur frequently it is important to see a homoeopath for constitutional treatment. Do not leave any ear condition untreated for too long because this can cause permanent hearing difficulties. If any obvious swelling is present seek urgent medical advice. Take the remedy in the 30c potency, 2–3 doses eight hours apart.

Aconite – *earache comes on suddenly after exposure to cold, dry winds*

Belladonna – *throbbing pain in the ear; ear looks red and feels hot*

Chamomilla – *pain is unbearable; earache at the time of teething; irritability; cheeks become red*

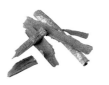

Ferrum phos – *use at the beginning of the inflammation; radiating and pulsating pains*

Hepar sulph – *yellow discharge from the ear that smells 'cheesy'; stitching pains; irritable and chilly*

Pulsatilla – *thick, yellow discharge from the ear; tearful and clingy; patient feels worse in warm conditions*

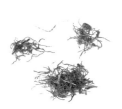

Silica – *offensive, thick, yellow-green discharge that can cause deafness*

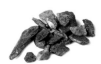

Eczema

Eczema, a form of dermatitis, is partially hereditary and can be exacerbated by allergens and common, everyday substances. The skin becomes dry, itchy and hot, causing extreme pain and bleeding in some cases, and it requires constitutional treatment from your homoeopath. The remedies below may help until you do so and should be taken in the 6c potency three times a day for 2–3 days.

Graphites – *eczema in folds of the skin; crusty, cracked skin; may ooze a honey-like discharge*

Sulphur – *skin looks unhealthy; red, hot itchy skin; patient may scratch until bleeding; aggravated by water and wool*

Eye injuries

Severe eye injuries must have urgent medical attention to prevent long-term damage in and around the eye area. Take the remedy in the 30c potency for one or two doses, each four hours apart. The remedy Silica can be taken in the 6x potency three times a day for 5 days.

Arnica – *injuries to the eye with bruising and haemorrhaging; good for shock*

Hamamelis – *for black eyes when the vision remains hazy*

Ledum – *for black eyes with puffiness and bruising; better for cold applications*

Silica – *helps to expel foreign bodies from the eye*

Eyestrain

Close or intensive work can over-strain the eyes, especially as so much work nowadays involves computers. Always make sure that you have sufficient light when working and that you rest your eyes frequently, occasionally focusing on objects that are further away. If symptoms persist, or if headaches are frequent, it is advisable to have your eyes tested. Take the remedy in the 6c potency three times a day until symptoms improve.

Ruta – *eyes feel hot and painful after close work or reading in dim light*

Fainting

Fainting occurs when there is a temporary lack of oxygen to the brain. If it becomes a common recurrence you should seek professional advice because there may be a particular prognosis that needs medical attention. Give one dose of the remedy in the 30c potency as required.

Chamomilla – *fainting as a result of intense pain*

Carbo veg – *fainting from poor circulation and lack of oxygen; patient has a desire to be fanned*

China – *fainting as a result of loss of fluids*

Ignatia – *fainting from emotional shock, grief or trauma*

Pulsatilla – *fainting in a hot, stuffy room*

Fever

Fevers actually benefit the body because they help to restore any imbalance resulting from illness. It is important, however, that the temperature during a fever does not run too high; seek professional advice immediately if it does. For mild fevers, the remedies below will help to speed up the recovery period. Plenty of fluids should be drunk to prevent dehydration, and sponging down with tepid water can also bring relief. Take the remedy in the 30c potency for 2–3 doses, two hours apart, or until symptoms improve.

Aconite – *sudden onset from cold, dry winds; anxiety and fear*

Arsenicum – *fluctuating temperature; feels cold externally, but burning inside; restless; thirsty for small sips of water*

Belladonna – *red face, dilated pupils and glassy eyes; patient feels restless and may start to hallucinate*

Eupatorium – *bones feel broken, chills start in the small of the back*

Ferrum phos – *flushed, hot face with a hammering headache; thirsty*

Gelsemium – *aching, shivering bones; exhausted and chilly; headache at the back of the head*

Merc sol – *sweating at night; sweat smells strongly and may stain the sheets; sensitive to temperature change*

Pulsatilla – *chilly, but worse for heat, with a need for fresh air; not thirsty; tearful*

Flatulence

This can be an uncomfortable condition, often food related and accompanied by bloating of the stomach. Take the remedy in the 6c potency as required.

Arg nit – *abdominal pain with gas and bloating; loud burping and passing of wind that brings no relief; anxiety*

Carbo veg – *bloating of the upper abdomen; foetid-smelling flatulence; burping relieves the symptoms; worse for eating rich, fatty foods*

China – *stomach feels tight, like a drum; not relieved by passing wind; worse when eating fruit*

Lycopodium – *gas and fullness in the stomach after eating even small amounts*

Mag phos – *cramping pains from the gas; better for warmth and massage*

Sulphur – *hot, with offensive smelling flatulence; rumbling stomach*

Fractures

These remedies will help the healing process once the fracture has been properly diagnosed. Take the remedy in the 6c potency – except for Calc phos which is 6x – twice a day for 2–3 weeks weeks.

Arnica – *bruising and shock after the accident*

Calc phos – *helps the fracture to heal more quickly*

Eupatorium – *aching pains deep inside the bone*

Hypericum – *shooting nerve pains*

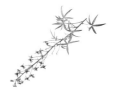

Gastroenteritis

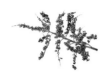

Stomach and intestines become inflamed due to bacteria, causing diarrhoea and vomiting. Sip water to prevent dehydration and take the remedy in the 6c potency three times a day for 2–3 days.

Arsenicum – *vomiting and diarrhoea with burning pains; restless and anxious; chilly with a desire for small sips of water*

Belladonna – *hot throbbing pains in the stomach with fever*

Bryonia – *movement feels unbearable; better for lying on the stomach; thirst for large quantities of water; desire to be alone with irritability*

Colocynth – *nausea and diarrhoea with agonizing cramping, twisting pains; better for hard pressure on the stomach*

Ipecac – *constant nausea aggravated by the thought or smell of food; diarrhoea and vomiting with no relief; tongue looks clean*

Mag phos – *violent cramping pains; better for warm applications or surroundings; bending forward and gentle massage help*

Nux vomica – *vomiting and diarrhoea a few hours after eating, with restricted feeling around the waist; irritable and moody*

Phosphorus – *burning pains in the stomach with a thirst for ice-cold water – vomiting occurs when this becomes warm in the stomach*

Podophyllum – *gushing and spluttering diarrhoea, with cramping pains; abdomen feels tender and sore*

Pulsatilla – *nausea and diarrhoea especially in children; the child is tearful and wants to be held*

Veratrum alb – *profuse diarrhoea and vomiting; chilly with a cold sweat; dizziness and fainting*

Grief

The death of a loved one, or the end of a relationship, is a painful time and people express their grief in many different ways. It is important to read the main Materia Medica section when selecting the remedy, and seeking advice from a homoeopath or a counsellor is highly recommended if it feels appropriate. Refer to the Useful Addresses section (page 138) for help in locating a homoeopath in your area. Take the remedy in the 30c potency: two doses eight hours apart.

Causticum – *suppressed grief; concerned for the welfare of others*

Ignatia – *emotional trauma; hysterical or silent; inability to accept what is happening*

Nat mur – *silent grief; emotions are shut out; patients feel they can cope when, in fact, they probably cannot*

Phos ac – *exhaustion after grief*

Growing pains

Growing pains felt by adolescents during growth spurts can be painful as the muscles and nerves go into spasm. The remedy below may help with calcium levels within the metabolism. Take the remedy in the 6x potency three times a day for ten days.

Calc phos – *gives essential nutrition during growth spurts*

Haemorrhoids

Haemorrhoids, also known as piles, are distended veins from the rectum, either internal or external. They will feel itchy and incredibly painful. If there is bleeding from the rectum it is important to establish the cause by seeking medical attention. Pregnancy or constipation can both be contributing factors. Take the remedy three times a day for 3–4 days in the 6c potency.

Calc fluor – *gives elasticity and tone to the blood vessel walls*

Hamamelis – *burning, itchy piles that feel raw and sore; piles bleed and protrude; sensation of a weight in the rectum*

Kali carb – *bleeding piles that feel as if a hot poker is in the anus; weakness*

Nit ac – *bleeding piles that itch and burn; the rectum feels torn when defecating*

Sulphur – *large piles that burn and smart; piles feel sore and tender*

Hangovers

Over indulgence of alcohol and other substances can often leave us worse for wear. Sufferers often feel tired, dehydrated and bloated. The

remedies below may help with any irritability, headaches, nausea and detoxification of the liver. Take the remedy in the 6c potency for 2–3 doses as needed.

Cocculus – *dizziness with a headache that is worse when moving; slow speech with delayed reactions*

Nat sulph – *liver feels sluggish; dull, heavy headache; aggravated by light and noise*

Nux vomica – *irritability; sensitive to light and noise; nausea and headache*

Hay fever

Hay fever is an allergic response, mainly triggered by pollens and grasses during the summer months. It affects the mucous membranes of the nose and eyes, causing discomfort to a huge proportion of the population year after year in the form of runny noses and sore eyes. The following remedies will help in an acute situation; however, constitutional treatment is advised. Take the remedy in the 6c potency three times a day; stop once the condition improves.

Allium cepa – *sneezing, together with burning discharge from the nose; bland tears from the eyes; feels worse entering a warm room*

Euphrasia – *eyes are burning, red and sore; acrid tears from the eyes with copious bland discharge from the nose that feels stuffed up during the night*

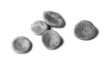

Headaches

There are several factors that contribute to headaches, most are obvious, such as stress, over-work or over-indulgence. Less obvious causes may be pollution or even food additives. If headaches are persistent or occur frequently, it is advisable to seek professional attention. Take remedies in the 6c potency three times a day for 1–2 days, or the 30c potency, in two doses, each four hours apart.

Aconite – *sudden, violent headache from cold, dry winds or a shock*

Arg nit – *congested headache from anxiety or mental effort; better for constriction around the head*

Belladonna – *throbbing, pounding headache; head feels hot; pupils dilated*

Bryonia – *severe bursting headache; patient is worse with any movement, especially sudden; feels better when lying alone in a dark room*

Calc phos – *school headaches from over-studying or worry; worse for fresh air*

Gelsemium – *pounding headache at the back of the head and neck that moves over the eyes*

Kali bich – *catarrhal headache; blurred vision with intolerance of noise and light*

Kali phos – *headaches from mental and physical exhaustion*

Nat mur – *hammering, bursting headaches; worse for the heat of the sun*

Nux vomica – *sick, toxic feeling; headache from over-indulgence; irritable, with sensitivity to light and noise*

Pulsatilla – *headache from being in a stuffy environment; better for fresh air; tearful*

Impetigo

Impetigo is a very contagious disease and care must be taken not to infect others. The skin is mainly affected on the hands and face, and the complaint usually results from contact with infected animals. Take the remedy in the 6c potency three times a day for 2–3 days.

Graphites – *crusty, cracked skin with a sticky discharge, rather like honey*

Merc sol – *open sores that ooze offensive pus*

Rhus tox – *blistering, itchy skin; burning sores*

Incontinence

Incontinence is a problem that is most commonly found in the elderly, during illness or after pregnancy, and it can be very distressing. Children do suffer, but this is referred to as bed wetting. Take the remedy in the 6c potency three times a day for 2–3 days. If there is no improvement, consult your homoeopath (see Useful Addresses – page 138).

Causticum – *paralysis of the bladder; involuntary urination when coughing, laughing or sneezing*

Sepia – *seepage of urine; feelings of tiredness, exhaustion and irritability*

Indigestion

Flatulence, heartburn and water brash (see Glossary – page 137) are all caused by indigestion. This, in turn, is usually caused by the consumption of overly rich or disagreeable foods, but stress and depression can give rise to it. If symptoms persist you should seek professional advice as there may be a more serious underlying cause. Take the remedy in the 30c potency in 1–2 doses.

Arsenicum – *burning pain in the stomach; irritable and restless; patient may feel thirsty*

Carbo veg – *flatulence and belching; stomach feels full and uncomfortable; worse from rich, fatty foods*

Nux vomica – *nausea and heartburn from over-indulgence; toxic irritability*

Pulsatilla – *nausea and distention from fatty foods; desire for fresh air; thirstlessness*

Injuries

First-aid remedies are useful to have in the home as many small injuries can be treated comfortably and easily. Seek urgent medical advice, however, especially in more serious situations such as unconsciousness or profuse bleeding. Bach's Rescue Remedy (see Glossary – page 134) can also be useful for any shock. Diluted Calendula and Hypericum tincture is useful for bathing cuts and grazes. Take the remedy in the 30c potency for 2–3 doses, four hours apart.

Arnica – *first remedy after injury for shock, bruising, haemorrhage and bleeding*

Hypericum – *injuries involving the nerves; sharp shooting pains; injury to the spine*

Ledum – *puncture wounds from rusty nails; crushed fingers; injured part is puffy but cold*

Nat sulph – *head injuries with memory loss; tinnitus and vertigo*

Opium – *head injuries with prolonged sleepiness*

Influenza

There are so many different strains of flu that a large amount of the population is regularly susceptible. This is particularly true with the elderly or those who feel run down and exhausted. The symptoms are more severe than those of a cold: fever, exhaustion and aching bones. Take the remedy in the 6c potency three times a day for 2–3 days.

Aconite – *sudden onset from cold winds; painful, dry cough; fever, restlessness and flushed face; anxiety*

Arsenicum – *cold but burning up inside; shivering and restless; sneezing with corrosive discharge*

Bryonia – *bursting headache and dry, painful cough; bones ache, worse with movement; desire to be alone and still; thirsty for great quantities of water*

Eupatorium – *bones feel broken; chills, sneezing and copious catarrh; eyes ache*

Gelsemium – *head and limbs feel heavy; shivering up and down the spine; drowsiness with little thirst*

Insomnia

Insomnia has many different causes and can come and go. As a rule, it is important to try to relax before bed in order to shut off the day's events. A warm bath containing the essential oil of lavender may help. If insomnia persists, it is advisable to visit a homoeopath for further treatment. Take one dose of the remedy in the 30c potency at bedtime and repeat if necessary.

Aconite – *fear or shock; frightening dreams*

Cocculus – *ailments from lack of sleep, nursing the sick or looking after a child*

Coffea – *mind unable to switch off; thoughts race round and round; restlessness*

Kali phos – *nervous exhaustion; patient is too tired to sleep*

Opium – *tiredness, but patient is unable to sleep due to over-sensitivity to noise*

Jet lag

Long-haul travel, which confuses the body's natural clock, can produce feelings of fatigue, otherwise known as jet lag. Take the remedy Arnica in the 30c potency every three hours during the flight. Take Kali phos in the 6x potency three times a day following arrival.

Arnica – *for shock to the system; enables the body to adapt to the new time and surroundings*

Kali phos – *for nervous exhaustion and fatigue after a long flight; unable to sleep*

Labour

It is often difficult to think about the remedies that can be of use during labour, but they can be very helpful if they are used in association with any medical assistance and birth plans that you choose. It is good to make your birth partner aware of the remedies and their uses well before you are due to give birth. There are many good labour kits available or, if you prefer to make your own, it may be useful to see your homoeopath first for guidance. Symptoms during labour may change and rapidly, you may, therefore, need to change the remedy frequently. Use the remedies in the 30c potency during labour.

Aconite – *fear and anxiety as labour begins*

Arnica – *for bruising, shock and haemorrhage*

Caulophyllum – *short, painful and ineffectual contractions; exhaustion*

Chamomilla – *screaming with the pain; abusive to those around them; can't bear to be touched*

China – *exhaustion after labour from loss of blood*

Coffea – *highly sensitive to the pain and noises; can become hysterical; may be unable to stop talking*

Gelsemium – *fear and anxiety; becomes rigid as labour progresses*

Kali carb – *labour ceases due to intense back pain*

Pulsatilla – *weak contractions; feel weepy and incapable; desire for fresh air*

Mastitis

Mastitis is an inflammation of the breasts most common in breast-feeding mothers, although some women suffer around their time of menstruation. It can be particularly painful, especially if abscesses form. Take the remedy in the 6c potency three times a day for 2–3 days.

Belladonna – *throbbing hot pain in the breasts with inflammation; breasts feel heavy and swollen*

Bryonia – *hot, hard breasts aggravated by movement; better for hard pressure*

Phytolacca – *stony hard breasts with tenderness; pain radiates from the breast to the back during breast-feeding*

Measles

This common childhood illness has an incubation period of 10–12 days and is most infectious before the rash starts. The child may have a fever, sore throat and eyes, and a cough, before the rash appears around the neck and behind the ears. White spots on the inside of the cheeks are often an initial indicator that the illness is measles. Take the remedy in the 6c potency three times a day for 3–4 days. Seek medical advice if you are worried about any symptoms or if the temperature is high and prolonged.

Aconite – *for the first stages: fever restlessness and anxiety; dry cough*

Belladonna – *hot, red face with fever and restlessness; dilated pupils; sore throat*

Bryonia – *dry, painful cough; rash is slow to appear; child is irritable and wants to be alone; light and noise aggravate; thirsty*

Euphrasia – *eyes are raw, sore and burning; tears scald the cheeks; runny nose; cough with a flushed face*

Pulsatilla – *bland or yellow catarrh with watery eyes; child is tearful and very clingy; better for fresh air*

Menstrual problems

Women experience many different physical and emotional symptoms before and during the time of their period. The remedies below may help with any discomfort experienced, and the Materia Medica section will also help. It is advisable to see a professional homoeopath for constitutional treatment to address emotional issues and to help re-balance the body. Professional advice is also recommended to diagnose any possible causes of discomfort, such as fibroids and cysts. Take the remedy in the 30c potency for 2–3 doses as needed.

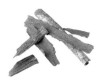

Aconite – *suppressed menstruation due to a fright or shock*

Apis – *stinging, burning pain in the ovaries*

Belladonna – *violent throbbing pains with a pulsating headache; hot, flushed face*

Caulophyllum – *scanty flow of blood; pains start in the small of the back; nausea and cramping pains*

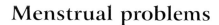

Chamomilla – *irritable and angry*

Colocynth – *twisting, cutting pains; better with pressure or lying on abdomen*

Ferrum phos – *painful periods; profuse bleeding; bright red blood*

Lachesis – *intense pain and discomfort before period; symptoms better for flow of blood; talkative*

Mag phos – *severe cramping pains; better for warmth, bending forwards and gentle massage*

Sepia – *heavy bleeding with bearing down pains; need to cross legs; irritability, especially with family members*

Veratrum alb – *cramping pains causing nausea, vomiting and diarrhoea; chilly with cold sweats*

Migraine

Migraines are intense headaches, and attacks can occur for a variety of reasons. Common symptoms are nausea, disturbed vision and acute light and noise sensitivity. It is advisable to see a homoeopath for constitutional treatment if they become a common occurrence. Stress is often a contributory factor, so relaxation methods, such as a massage, may help. For an acute situation take the remedy in the 6c or 30c potency for 1–2 doses as needed. Stop on improvement.

Belladonna – *pounding, throbbing migraine; hot, flushed face with glassy eyes; head needs to be held; better when head is bent backwards*

Bryonia – *severe bursting headache; all movement aggravates; desire to be in a dark room, alone, silent; nausea and vomiting*

Gelsemium – *headache starts at the back of the head and moves over the eyes; head feels heavy and dull, as if a band is around the head; better for urinating*

Kali bich – *catarrhal headache with blurred vision; pain can be pinpointed*

Nux vomica – *toxic headache, aggravated by stimulants; nausea and vomiting; irritable*

Pulsatilla – *migraine from eating fatty foods, digestive and menstrual disorders; worse in a warm, stuffy room; tearful*

Morning sickness

Many women experience sickness in the first few months of pregnancy, which is often triggered by certain foods or smells. The feelings of nausea and actual vomiting itself are not just confined to the morning, although they may be more common at that time of day. The symptoms do tend to subside after the third month but, if this is not the case, it is advisable to see your homoeopath. Take the remedy in the 6c potency for 1–2 doses when needed.

Cocculus – *dizziness with nausea; smell and thought of food brings on vomiting; worse for moving about*

Ipecac – *constant nausea, not relieved by vomiting; clean tongue with lack of thirst*

Nux vomica – *nausea; better for vomiting*

and belching; heartburn; indigestion;
irritability

Pulsatilla – *nausea from fatty foods with little vomiting; worse in warm rooms; lack of thirst*

Sepia – *exhaustion; nausea aggravated by the thought or smell of food, but relieved by eating*

Mouth ulcers

Mouth ulcers are often associated with debility, and this should be addressed as part of the treatment. If ulcers occur frequently it is advisable to see your homoeopath for constitutional treatment. Take the remedy in the 6c potency three times a day for 2–3 days.

Merc sol – *ulceration with copious saliva; tongue flabby; metallic taste in the mouth*

Mumps

This infectious childhood illness affects the glands, which become swollen and tender along the jaw line. Fever and a sore throat are the first indicators. Take the remedy in the 30c potency for 2–3 doses.

Aconite – *first stages with sore throat; anxiety and fever*

Apis – *hot; puffiness with stinging pains; lack of thirst*

Belladonna – *throbbing pains with heat and swelling; difficulty in swallowing; fever and glassy eyes*

Merc sol – *swollen glands with stitching pains to the ear on swallowing; breath smells*

Pulsatilla – *swollen glands; child tearful and clingy; desire for fresh air*

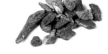

Nausea

Pregnancy, digestive disturbances and intense pain can all cause nausea. If you are uncertain as to the cause of your sickness, or your symptoms persist, it is advisable to seek professional advice from your homoeopath or medical practitioner. For mild cases, try one of the appropriate remedies below in the 6c potency for 1–2 doses.

Cocculus – *dizziness with nausea; worse for travelling or any movement*

Ipecac – *constant nausea; not relieved by vomiting*

Nux vomica – *nausea from excessive stimulants; better for vomiting*

Kali phos – *nausea when nervous; better for nibbling small amounts of food*

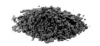

Phosphorus – *nausea after an anaesthetic*

Neuralgia

Neuralgia is a painful inflammation of the nerves, especially in the face or back. Take the remedy in the 6c potency three times a day for 2–3 days, and if the symptoms persist see your homoeopath.

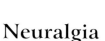

Colocynth – *shooting pains; better for lying on the painful side*

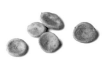

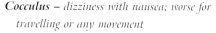

Hypericum – *sharp, shooting pains; severe nerve pain*

Kali phos – *lightning-like pains shooting along the nerves*

Mag Phos – *shooting pains along the spine; better for warmth*

Nosebleeds

Nosebleeds usually occur because of accidents or injuries. If spontaneous nosebleeds are common seek professional advice. Take the remedy in the 6c or 30c potency for 2–3 doses.

Aconite – *nosebleed starts after a shock or fright; bright red blood*

Arnica – *for nosebleeds after a blow, injury or accident*

Ferrum phos – *bright red blood; most common in children*

Hamamelis – *spontaneous or after an accident; bleeding takes a long time to stop*

Phosphorus – *profuse bleeding; bright red and slow to stop*

Operations

The remedies below will help to support the body during this traumatic time, expediting the healing process. Arnica is particularly useful and can be taken before the operation to limit the amount of bruising and shock. Take any remedy in the 30c potency for 2–3 doses as needed.

Arg nit – *anxiety and apprehension before an operation*

Arnica – *shock, bruising and haemorrhage*

Bellis perennis – *deep internal bruising; post-operative pain*

Phosphorus – *nausea and vomiting after the anaesthetic*

Staphysagria – *stinging and smarting pains; body feels invaded*

Palpitations

Palpitations usually result from shock, worry or excitement that causes the heart to beat faster. The remedies below may help for mild palpitations, but it is useful to read the Materia Medica section to confirm your choice. It is always important to seek professional advice if the palpitations occur frequently or if there are sudden changes to your regular heartbeat. Take the remedy in the 6c potency as needed.

Aconite – *pounding heart from shock or fright*

Aurum – *weight around the heart; heart thumps violently; breathlessness*

Lachesis – *circulation disturbed; flushed face with hot flushes and high blood pressure; talkative and excited*

Period pains

see Menstrual problems

Perspiration

Perspiration is necessary for temperature regulation and for the elimination of unwanted toxins from the body. Despite our need to feel clean and to smell appealing to ourselves and other people, especially in social situations, suppressing perspiration through the use of anti-perspirants is not always advisable. The remedies below offer a more healthy alternative for everyday use. Excessive sweating, if not from an obvious cause, should be addressed by seeking professional advice. Take the remedy in the 30c potency for 2–3 doses.

Calc carb – *sweaty, flabby babies; sweat may smell sour*

Merc sol – *offensive smelling sweat that stains clothes and bedding*

Silica – *head and face will sweat in children; smelly feet*

Pregnancy

The remedies below may help for some situations that arise during pregnancy. You may decide to start using them at an even earlier stage of pregnancy to enhance the health of your unborn baby. In all cases, it is important to have the advice of a professional homoeopath during this time. The remedies below also help with changes in your body, such as stretch marks and stress to the joints

and muscles. See also Labour and Morning sickness for further remedies. In the cases of Bellis perennis and Pulsatilla, take the remedy in the 30c potency for 1–2 doses. For Calc fluor and Ferrum phos take the remedy in the 6x potency twice a day for ten days.

Bellis perennis – *problems walking from strained abdominal muscles; bruising from baby kicking*

Calc fluor – *helps with the elasticity of the skin, preventing stretch marks; tones the pelvic area*

Ferrum phos – *for anaemia during pregnancy; helps with the absorption of iron*

Pulsatilla – *tearful and needy, feel they can't cope; may help the baby turn around if in breech position*

Rheumatism

The inflammation of the connective tissues surrounding muscles or tendons can cause the muscles to tighten, which may, in turn, deform the joints. The pains move around the body, mainly emanating from the muscles, tendons and ligaments. Treatment from a professional medical practitioner is important, but the remedies below may give some relief. Take the remedy in the 6c potency three times a day for 4–5 days.

Arnica – *bruised, aching limbs that feel worse from exercise and over-straining*

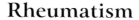

127

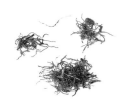

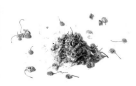

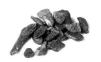

Bryonia *– painful, swollen joints that are worse for any movement; better for lying still on the painful part*

Caulophyllum *– drawing pains in the smaller joints that seem to fly around the body*

Ferrum phos *– any sudden inflammation of the joints*

Kali bich *– red hot, swollen joints associated with catarrhal and digestive problems*

Ledum *– stiff burning pains; better with any cold applications*

Rhus tox *– swelling and stiffness; parts feel bruised and numb; worse on first moving; better with continuous movement; aggravated by damp weather*

Scabies

Scabies is an uncomfortable skin condition, causing immense itching and irritation. It is the result of mites that burrow into the skin. Any warmth, especially at night, will aggravate the itching, and a rash will appear, although not above the neckline. Take the remedy in the 6c potency three times a day for 5 days.

Sulphur *– skin is intolerably itchy and hot; unhealthy-looking skin*

Sciatica

Sciatica involves pain in the lower back that travels down the sciatic nerve, affecting the thighs, knees and sometimes even the feet. Take the remedy in the 6c potency three times a day for 2–3 days. Other holistic treatments such as Acupuncture and Osteopathy (see Glossary – pages 134 and 136 respectively) may also help to relieve the condition.

Colocynth *– shooting pains; better for lying on the affected side*

Hypericum *– violent, shooting, tearing nerve pains*

Kali phos *– lightning-like pains*

Mag phos *– sharp, shooting, spasmodic pain; better for warmth and massage*

Ruta *– pains are worse going up the stairs and in the evening, when lying down*

Shingles

Shingles, otherwise known as *Herpes zoster*, is a viral infection related to chicken pox. The initial fever, which usually lasts for a few days, is followed by a red rash that forms blisters at the nerve-endings, causing intense, long-lasting pain, itching and burning. Debility is often a cause. Take the remedy in the 6c potency, or 6x for Kali phos, three times a day for one week.

Arsenicum *– burning pains; better for warmth; restlessness and anxiety*

Colocynth *– shooting pains; better for lying on the affected side*

Kali phos *– lightning-like pains along the nerves*

Rhus tox *– intensely itchy, fluid-filled blisters*

Shock

Shock can be a potentially serious condition, putting great strain on the physical body. It can affect blood pressure and cause fainting, irregular breathing patterns and generally upset your well-being. If you are worried about the symptoms you are suffering, you must seek medical attention. However, the remedies below may help in acute situations and prevent further treatment being necessary. Take the remedy in the 30c potency, in 1–2 doses, as needed. Bach's Rescue Remedy (see Glossary – page 134) is also useful in cases of shock.

Aconite – *shock and fear; panic may last long after the initial trauma*

Arnica – *shock after injury or accident; patient may say they are well, when this is not the case*

Chamomilla – *shock from pain; possible hysteria*

China – *shock after loss of blood*

Ignatia – *shock from grief and trauma; fainting*

Opium – *withdrawal after grief; trauma and shock*

Sinusitis

Sinusitis occurs when the sinus cavities become inflamed, increasing the production of mucus. Chronic sinusitis should be treated constitutionally by a professional

homoeopath. It is often helpful to limit your dairy product intake as this can increase the mucus production. Take the remedy in the 6c potency three times a day for 3–4 days.

Bryonia – *bursting frontal headache, with dryness of the nasal passages*

Kali bich – *stuffed up feeling at the root of the nose; thick, stringy mucus comes out in a rope-like fashion*

Merc sol – *infected sinuses; ulceration in the nose; yellow-green mucus; nasty taste in the mouth*

Pulsatilla – *thick, yellow discharge; nose stuffed up at night, flows during the day; better in fresh air*

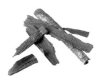

Sore throat

Sore throats are often the first sign of illness or being run down. Treatment at this early stage can often prevent the illness from going any further or help speed up the healing process. Take the remedy in the 6c potency three times a day until symptoms improve, or in the 30c potency for 2–3 doses.

Aconite – *sudden sore throat from cold, dry winds; inflamed or red-raw sore throat; burning thirst and fever*

Belladonna – *dry, inflamed, burning throat; red and swollen tonsils; fever*

Calc phos – *recurrent sore throats with swollen tonsils and glands*

Cantharis – *intense burning in the throat; thirsty but throat is too painful to drink; touching the larynx creates spasms*

Ferrum phos – *beginning of inflammation with hoarse voice; redness and ulceration*

Hepar sulph – *painful stitching and splinter-like pains; pain extends to ears when swallowing*

Lachesis – *sensation of lump in the throat; unable to eat or drink due to intense pain*

Merc sol – *ulceration and suppuration of the throat and tonsils; stitching pains which extend to the ears; foul taste in the mouth; smelly breath*

Nit ac – *sensation of a fish bone in the throat; splinter-like pain; ulceration of the throat; smelly breath*

Phytolacca – *recurrent tonsillitis; dark red tonsils covered with white spots; sensation of hot lump in the throat; pain extends to ears*

Splinters

Foreign bodies, such as shafts of wood or glass, that lodge under the surface of the skin usually push themselves out. The remedies below may help speed up this process. Bathing the remedy in the diluted tincture of Calendula and Hypericum (see table – page 14) may help prevent any infection. Take the remedy in the 6x potency three times a day for 3–4 days for the remedy Silica and in the 30c potency for Hypericum for 2–3 doses.

Hypericum – *painful shooting pains*

Silica – *helps eliminate foreign bodies*

Sprains and strains

Injury to the tendons and ligaments can be very painful, and it is important to rule out the possibility of a fracture. Support bandages and limited use of the affected part are most beneficial. Take the remedy in the 6c potency three times a day for 3–4 days.

Arnica – *parts feel sore and bruised with swelling after over-exertion or accidents*

Bellis perennis – *deep, bruised soreness; straining of abdominal wall during pregnancy*

Bryonia – *parts feel swollen and sore; worse for any movement; must keep part still; better when lying on painful part*

Calc fluor – *over-stretched ligaments and tendons; better for movement; lower back pain*

Hypericum – *shooting nerve pains; back pain from a fall on the coccyx*

Rhus tox – *stiff, sore, swollen joints; feels worse on first movement, but better for continuous movement*

Ruta – *painful tendons and ligaments; feels worse for moving too much*

Stretch marks

Fluctuations in body weight and pregnancy often lead to stretch marks. The use of wheatgerm oil is beneficial for the elasticity of the skin due to its high vitamin E content. Take the remedy in the 6x potency twice a day for ten days.

Calc fluor – *helps give tone and elasticity*

Styes

Styes are infected and swollen pimples or boils that appear on the margins of the eyelid around the eyelashes. Although they are very painful, there is no actual harm to the eyeball or to the patient's vision. Take the remedy three times a day in the 6c potency for 3–4 days.

Apis – *hot, fiery, stinging pains; redness and swelling*

Hepar sulph – *splinter-like pains; very sensitive to touch*

Silica – *helps speed up healing process; expels any lingering discharge*

Staphysagria – *stinging, smarting pain; recurrent styes*

Sunburn

Staying out in the sun, wherever you live, can inflict long-lasting damage to your body. Protection is always better than cure and far less painful! If the sunburn is severe it is important to seek medical attention. Remember to drink plenty of fluids to prevent dehydration. In addition, a sufferer may go into a state of shock. (See also Shock for extra help with any treatment). Take the remedy in the 6c potency three times a day for 2–3 days.

Belladonna – *red, dry, hot skin; bursting, throbbing headache*

Nat mur – *intense, migraine-like headache*

Teething

Teething can be a distressing time for both child and parent. Irritability, fever and diarrhoea can all be symptomatic. Take the remedy in the 6c potency as needed.

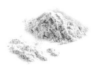

Calc carb – *teething can be delayed and difficult; babies tend to be flabby, hot and sweaty*

Calc phos – *promotes strong teeth; good for soft teeth and painful gums; may be accompanied by green diarrhoea*

Chamomilla – *red, painful gums; one cheek is red and the other pale; child is very irritable; stools have the appearance of chopped spinach*

Ferrum phos – *redness and inflammation with a slight fever*

Tonsillitis

see Sore throat

Toothache

Pain in teeth and gums can be caused by decay, but the stresses of everyday life may also be to blame. Take the remedy in the 30c potency for two to three doses. Use the remedy Calc fluor in the 6x potency twice a day for ten days. If symptoms persist see your dentist.

Arnica – *bruised, sore sensation after injury or a trip to the dentist; helps to stop bleeding after a tooth extraction*

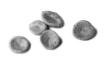

Calc fluor – *supports decaying teeth*

Coffea – *nerve pain that feels better with any cold-water applications*

Ferrum phos – *inflammation and redness around the gums*

Hepar sulph – *tooth abscess; pus is forming; area feels tender and sore*

Hypericum – *shooting nerve pain*

Kali phos – *nagging toothache in decayed or filled teeth*

Mag phos – *sharp, shooting nerve pains; relieved by warmth*

Silica – *weakened enamel; sore abscesses and boils*

Travel sickness

Many people find different kinds of motion and movement aggravating to the point of nausea and vomiting. Chewing ginger or drinking ginger tea can sometimes relieve the symptoms. Take the remedy below in the 6c potency as needed.

Cocculus – *dizziness, vertigo, nausea and vomiting from travelling; watching moving objects intensifies the symptoms*

Varicose veins

Varicose veins are swollen, distended veins that are often a sign of poor circulation, lack of exercise, a sedentary job or extra abdominal weight, such as in pregnancy, when there is added pressure on the internal organs. There may also be hereditary factors to take into account. Take the remedy in the 6c potency three times a day for 2–3 days. Calc fluor should be taken in the 6x potency three times a day for ten days.

Bellis perennis – *varicose veins feel squeezed, bruised and sore*

Calc fluor – *varicose veins due to loss of tone in the blood vessel walls*

Carbo veg – *poor circulation; varicose veins have a tendency to ulcerate*

Hamamelis – *painful varicose veins that are knotty-hard and feel full*

Lachesis – *painful varicose veins with a tendency to ulcerate*

Vomiting

If vomiting is persistent it is advisable to seek professional advice, especially with young children. Try to drink plenty of fluids to prevent dehydration. Take the remedy in the 6c or 30c potency for 2–3 doses as needed.

Arsenicum – *burning pains in the stomach; restless, chilly, thirsty for small sips*

Bryonia – *thirsty for large quantities of water; patient needs to be still and quiet with no distraction; vomiting from headaches*

Cocculus – *vomiting from travelling; griping pains with dizziness; aversion to food or drink*

Ipecac – *constant nausea and vomiting; vomiting does not relieve the symptoms*

Nux vomica – *vomiting from over-indulgence in stimulants; irritability*

Phosphorus – *thirst for large quantities of cold water that is vomited as soon as it becomes warm in the stomach; burning pains*

Podophyllum – *profuse, watery vomit accompanied by spluttering diarrhoea*

Pulsatilla – *vomiting from eating fatty foods; better for fresh air*

Veratrum alb – *vomiting at the same time as the diarrhoea; patient feels cold and has a cold sweat; desire for ice cubes*

Warts and verrucae

Constitutional treatment from a professional homoeopath is recommended for the treatment of warts and verrucae, especially if they reoccur frequently. Take the remedy in the 6c potency three times a day for seven days.

Causticum – *warts found mainly on the hands, face and lids of the eyes*

Nit ac – *jagged warts that bleed easily*

Whooping cough

These remedies may be used as a support in conjunction with medical treatment, as this childhood illness can be very serious. The first signs are usually a sore throat, cold and fever, which then develop into the distinctive whooping, barking cough, causing the child to gasp for air. Take 2–3 doses of the 30c potency eight hours apart, or the 6c potency three times a day for five days.

Bryonia – *very hard, painful cough; must hold the chest to restrict the movement; child wants to be left alone and be still*

Carbo veg – *child craves fresh air and may turn blue from the coughing fit; strong feelings of suffocation; exhaustion*

Drosera – *deep, hollow, barking cough; comes in fits and leads to vomiting; fear of suffocation*

Ipecac – *incessant cough; child becomes rigid, and develops a red or blue face with vomiting*

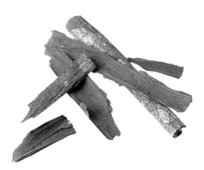

Glossary

Acupuncture

A traditional form of Chinese healing that uses needles to puncture the skin at specified points – 'acupoints' – in order to cure illness or relieve symptoms and promote healing.

Acute illness

This refers to self-limiting illnesses that, given time, will clear up of their own accord, such as colds, flu or measles. Some acute illnesses – pneumonia, for example – can be fatal. There tends to be three stages that a patient goes through: incubation, when symptoms are present but not obvious; illness, when symptoms are obvious; and finally, convalescence.

Affinity

When the characteristics of a remedy taken by a healthy person reflect strongly those of the specified ailment.

Ailment

Another name for 'illness'.

Antidote

A substance that reduces the effectiveness of a homoeopathic remedy, in some cases negating it all together. Drinking coffee can sometimes have this effect.

Allopathy

Another word for conventional medicine, coined by Hahnemann to distinguish it from homoeopathy. It comes from the Greek words *allo* meaning 'opposite', and *pathos* meaning 'suffering'.

Bach's Rescue Remedy

This is a combination of five flowers – cherry plum, clematis, impatiens, rock rose and Star of Bethlehem – originally used by Dr Edward Bach in the early twentieth century to combat negative emotional states. It can be used in any emergency situation to ease anxiety, fear or shock.

Case taking

The collection of all the relevant symptoms of a patient, so that an accurate diagnosis can be made and the correct remedy prescribed.

Centesimal scale

The dilution of the mother tincture by one part of the tincture to 99 parts of alcohol, indicated in the dosage by the letter 'c'. See also Decimal scale.

Chronic illness

This refers to any long term, deep-seated illness that endures for a long, often unpredictable period of time, sometimes with changing symptom patterns. Acute illnesses can develop into chronic ones, which is why it is always important to consult a qualified homoeopath. Cancer and arthritis are examples of chronic illnesses.

Common symptoms
Symptoms that are commonly found in a specific illness – helping to identify that illness – such as spots in chicken pox.

Constitution
The condition of a person's health at any particular time, often assessed by observation alone, notwithstanding genetic factors inherited through the family.

Constitutional remedy
A homoeopathic remedy that helps re-balance the overall constitution of a patient, including their mental, emotional and physical well-being. Constitutional remedies are chosen by examing the person as a whole, and are best prescribed by a qualified homoeopath.

Convalescence
The period following an illness when the patient's system is weakened while the body and the remedy work to restore full health –

that is, a time for re-balancing the constitution.

Debility
A weakened state during and following illness.

Decimal scale
The dilution of the mother tincture by one part of the tincture to ten parts of alcohol, symbolized by the use of the letter 'x' in the dosage. See also Centesimal scale.

Differentiate
To look at the differences between two remedy pictures, bearing in mind the patient's symptoms, in order to make the most suitable choice.

Emotional picture
The collection of the emotional symptoms, feelings and moods of a person. Also used when referring to the emotional symptoms that are found within a remedy.

Essence
The overall sense or meaning of a particular remedy.

Expectoration
The coughing or spitting out of phlegm from the chest or lungs.

Homoeopathic aggravation

A temporary worsening of the symptoms after taking a certain homoeopathic remedy. This most often occurs after taking a constitutional remedy.

Key note

A very important and specific symptom of a homoeopathic remedy.

Law of Similars

Hahnemann's first law in homoeopathy, stating that a substance can cure a sick person of the symptoms that it produces in a healthy person: 'Like cures like.'

Localized symptoms

Symptoms that occur in limited and specific areas of the body.

Main indications

The most common symptoms – mental, emotional and physical – of a remedy.

Maintaining cause

Something that causes constant stress on the body, making it difficult for the remedy to have any curative action.

Materia Medica

The collective descriptions of all the remedy pictures, usually written down in alphabetical order.

Mental symptoms

How the thinking process is affected – e.g., concentration, memory etc.

Miasm

Comes from the Greek word *miasma* meaning 'pollution'. It is a word used by homoeopaths to describe an obstacle to getting better – either through heredity or from a previous illness.

Minimum dose

The potentization – i.e., establishing the correct strength – of a remedy that cures without giving rise to side effects.

Modalities

Factors that makes symptoms either better or worse.

Mother tincture

This is the starting material for a homoeopathic remedy. The original substance is taken and steeped in alcohol for a long period of time. This, in turn, is then used for the process of dilution and succussion.

Nosode

A homoeopathic remedy made from diseased tissue – i.e., a small pox vesicle.

Osteopathy

This is a system of treatment that involves spinal manipulation and massage to relieve back pain.

Picture

The overall symptoms of a person or remedy.

Potency

This describes the strength of the remedy and is determined by how many times it has been diluted and shaken.

Proving

The method used for establishing the healing properties of a remedy. This is achieved by administering substances to healthy patients under controlled conditions and observing their reactions.

Remedy

The name given to a homoeopathic medicine.

Repertory

Any book, or section of a book, used by homoeopaths that contains an index of symptoms followed by a list of all the remedies associated with these symptoms, and used in conjunction with the Materia Medica.

Sac lac

The name given to the pill used as a carrier for the remedy, made from sugar and milk.

Similimum

The remedy picture that most closely matches the symptom picture of the patient.

Succussion

This refers to the shaking process used after the dilution of the mother tincture in order to release the energy of the raw material.

Suppression

The masking of symptoms that subsequently drives the illness further into the body.

Susceptibility

The level to which someone is prone to certain illnesses.

Symptoms

Any change to a person's normal, healthy state on an emotional, mental and physical level.

Symptom picture

The collection of all the symptoms of one particular person. This is then used to determine which remedy should be used.

Vital force

The name Hahnemann used for the energy that exists within all living things. He claimed that vital force needs to be balanced for us to remain healthy.

Water brash

A reflex action causing excessive acid fluids from the stomach to go into the mouth.

Useful Addresses

Societies & Institutes

UK

The Society of Homoeopaths
4a Artizan Road, Northampton, NN1 4HU
Tel: (01604) 621400
Fax: (01604) 622622
E-mail: info@homeopathy-soh.org
Web site:
http://www.homeopathy-soh.org

The British Homoeopathic Association
27a Devonshire Street, London,
WC1N 3HZ
Tel: (020) 7935 2163
E-mail: brithom@talk21.com
Web site: http://www.nhsconfed\bha

Faculty of Homoeopathy
The Royal Homoeopathic Hospital,
Great Ormond Street, London, WC1N 3HR
Tel: (020) 7837 8833
Fax: (020) 7833 7229

Council for Complementary and Alternative Medicine
63 Jeddo Road, London, W12 6HQ
Tel: (020) 8735 0632

British Complementary Medical Association
Kensington House, 33 Imperial Square,
Cheltenham, Gloucestershire, GL50 1QZ
Tel: (0116) 282 5511
Fax: (0116) 227765

AUSTRALIA

Australian Association of Professional Homoeopaths
80 Essenden Road, Anstead, Queensland 4070
Tel: (617) 320 26517
E-mail: ann_tacey@telstra.easymail.com.au

Australian Homoeopathic Association
Federal Body, C/- 65 Brosely Road, Toowong,
Queensland 4068
Tel: (617) 337 17245

Australian Council of Homoeopathy
P.O. Box 494, Lindfield,
New South Wales 2070
Tel: (612) 980 96703

Homoeopathic Education and Research Association
1st Floor, 151 Union Street, Windsor,
Victoria 3181
Tel: (613) 952 12779

CANADA

Ontario Homeopathic Association
P.O. Box 258, Station P, Toronto,
Ontario, M5S 2S7
Tel: (416) 488 9685 / (416) 222 2995
E-mail: root@ontariohomeopath.com
Web site: http://www.ontariohomeopath.com

Homeopathic College of Canada
280 Eglinton Avenue East, Toronto,
Ontario, MP4 1L4
Tel: (416) 481 8816
E-mail: info@homeopathy.edu

Syndicat professionel des homéopathes du Quebec
1600 de Lorimier, Suite 382, Montréal,
Quebec, H2K 3W5
Tel: (514) 525 2037
Fax: (514) 525 1299
E-mail: sphq@total.net

Homoeopathic Suppliers

UK

Ainsworth's Homoeopathic Pharmacy
38 New Cavendish Street, London, W1M 7LH
Tel: (020) 7935 5330
Fax: (020) 7486 4313
E-mail: ainshom@msn.com

Helios Homoeopathic Pharmacy
89-97 Camden Road, Royal Tunbridge Wells,
Kent, TN1 2QR
Tel: (01892) 536393 / 537254
Fax: (01892) 546850
E-mail: pharmacy@helios.co.uk

Weleda UK Ltd
Heanor Road, Ilkeston, Derbyshire, DE/ 8DR
Tel: (020) 7629 3118
Fax: (020) 7495 0018
E-mail: weledauk@compuserve.com
Web site: http://www.weleda.co.uk

AUSTRALIA

Brauer Biotherapies
Tanunda, South Australia 5352
Tel: (618) 8563 2932

Pharmaceutical Plant Company
24 London Drive, Bayswater, Victoria 3153
Tel: (613) 9762 3777

CANADA

Bach-Karooch
P.O.Box 2465, Peterborough, Ontario, K9J 7Y8
Tel: (705) 749 1894
Fax: (705) 749 0275
E-mail: wildboy@peterboro.net

Neal's Yard Remedies
NYR homoeopathic products can be obtained
in many parts of the world. Contact the UK
head office for details of your nearest outlet:

Head Office: 26-34 Ingate Place, London,
SW8 3NS *Tel:* (020) 7498 1686
Fax: (020) 7498 2505

Mail Order: 29 John Dalton Street Manchester,
M2 6DS *Tel:* (0161) 831 7875
Fax: (0161) 835 9322

Customer Services: Tel: (020) 7627 1949

Neal's Yard Remedies' outlets worldwide:
UK
15 Neal's Yard, Covent Garden, London, WC2H
9DP *Tel:* (020) 7379 7222

Chelsea Farmers Market, Sydney Street,
London, SW3 6NR *Tel:* (020) 7351 6380

9 Elgin Crescent, London, W11 2JA
Tel: (020) 7727 3998

68 Chalk Farm Road, Camden, London,
NW1 8AN *Tel:* (020) 7284 2039

2a Kensington Gardens, Brighton,
East Sussex, BN1 4AL *Tel:* (01273) 601464

126 Whiteladies Road, Clifton, Bristol, BS8 2RP
Tel: (0117) 946 6034

The Glades Shopping Centre, Bromley, Kent,
BR1 1DD *Tel:* (020) 8313 9898

23–25 Morgan Arcade, Cardiff, CF1 2AF
Tel: (029) 2023 5721

9 Rotunda Terrace, Montpellier Street,
Cheltenham, GL50 1SX *Tel:* (01242 522136)

46a George Street, Edinburgh, EH2 2LE
Tel: (0131) 226 3223

29 John Dalton Street, Manchester,
M2 6DS *Tel:* (0161) 831 7875

19 Central Arcade, Newcastle-Upon-Tyne,
NE1 5BQ *Tel:* (0191) 232 2525

26 Lower Goat Lane, Norwich, NR2 1EL
Tel: (01603) 766681

5 Golden Cross, Cornmarket Street, Oxford,
OX1 3EU *Tel:* (01865) 2454436

South America
Rua Melo Alves 383, Jardins, Sao Paulo, CEP
01417 010, Brazil

Japan
4-9-3 Jingumae, Shibuya-ku, Tokyo 150-000

Venus Fort 2F, Palette Town, 1 Aomi Koto-ku,
Tokyo 135-0064

Queen's East 2F, 2-3-2 Minatomirai, Nishi-ku,
Yokahama, Kanagawa Pre. 220

Super Brand City, 3-1 Shimokawabata-cho,
Hakata-ku, Fukuoka City, Fukuota 812 0027

USA
79 East Putnam Avenue, Greenwich,
Connecticut, CT 06830-5644

Further Reading

Coulter, C. R., *Portraits of Homoeopathic Medicines.* North Atlantic Books, 1988

Gibson, Dr D., *Studies of Homoeopathic Remedies.* Beaconsfield Publishers, 1991

Grieve, M., *A Modern Herbal.* Tiger Books International, 1994

Hamilton, E., *The Flora Homoeopathica.* B. Jain Publishers Pvt. Ltd., 1995

Kent, Dr J. T., *Lectures on Homoeopathic Philosophy.* Insight Editions, 1985

Kent, Dr J. T., *Materia Medica of Homoeopathic Remedies.* Homoeopathic Book Service, 1989

Phatak, Dr S. R., *Materia Medica of Homoeopathic Medicine.* Indian Books & A Periodicals Syndicate, 1982

Scholten, J., *Homoeopathy and Minerals.* Stichting Alonnissos, 1993

Shepherd, D., *A Physicians Posy.* Health Science Press, 1981

Tyler, M. L., *Homoeopathic Drug Pictures.* B. Jain Publishers Ltd., 1997

Vermeulen, F., *Concordant Materia Medica.* Merlijn Publishers, 1994

Vermeulen, F., *Synoptic Materia Medica.* Merlijn Publishers, 1993

Vithoulkhas, G., *Homoeopathy – Medicine of the New Man.* Thorsons, 1979

Index